The Medicalization
of Everyday Life

Thomas Szasz

The Medicalization *of* Everyday Life

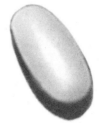

S E L E C T E D   E S S A Y S

Syracuse University Press

Syracuse University Press
Syracuse, New York 13244-5160

The paper used in this publication meets the minimum requirements
of American National Standard for Information Sciences—Permanence
of Paper for Printed Library Materials, ANSI Z39.48-1984.∞™

For a listing of books published and distributed by Syracuse University Press,
visit our Web site at SyracuseUniversityPress.syr.edu.

ISBN-13: 978-0-8156-0867-7
ISBN-10: 0-8156-0867-5

LIBRARY OF CONGRESS CATALOGING-IN-PUBLICATION DATA

Szasz, Thomas Stephen, 1920–
The medicalization of everyday life : selected essays / Thomas Szasz. — 1st ed.
p. ; cm.
Selection of essays presented or published between 1972 and 2006.
Includes bibliographical references and index.
ISBN-13: 978-0-8156-0867-7 (pbk. : alk. paper)   ISBN-10: 0-8156-0867-5 (pbk. : alk. paper)
1. Mental illness—Classification—Social aspects. 2. Mental illness—Diagnosis—Social aspects.
3. Diseases—Classification—Social aspects. 4. Psychiatry—Moral and ethical aspects.
5. Medical ethics. I. Title.
[DNLM: 1. Psychiatry—ethics—United States—Collected Works. 2. Health Policy—
United States—Collected Works. 3. Health Services Misuse—United States—Collected Works.
4. Psychotherapy—ethics—United States—Collected Works. WM 62 S996m 2007]
RC455.2.C4S93 2007
306.4'61—dc22   2007022129

Contents

Preface

WHEN I USE MEDICAL TERMS such as "diagnosis," "disease," and "treatment" in reference to psychiatry or psychoanalysis, it is with the understanding that we are not dealing with real, literal diagnoses, diseases, or treatments. We are dealing with the *metaphorical uses of these terms*. However, this medicalized idiom is such an integral part of our contemporary culture that the terms are accepted on face value, as *literal* diagnoses, diseases, and treatments. Indeed, it is socially improper—embarrassing, offensive, insulting—to reassert their metaphorical character. Still worse is calling attention to the practical—legal and medical—consequences that follow, linguistically and logically, from identifying and "treating" nondiseases as diseases. My writings about mental illness and psychiatry reflect my insistence on making this simple but fundamental distinction.

Calling this distinction "simple" is not the same as saying that it is easy to grasp or accept. Countless writers have remarked on the remarkable properties of language and on the profound connections between language, thought, religion, science, and social existence in general. One of the most elegant and lucid statements that I have come across is the following:

> Metaphors are a valuable literary device. They enrich language by making it dramatic and colorful, rendering abstract concepts concrete, condensing complex concepts into a few words, and unleashing creative and analogical insights. But their uncritical use can lead to confusion and distortion. At its heart, metaphor compares two or more things that are not, in fact, identical. A metaphor's literal meaning is used non-literally in a comparison with its subject. While the comparison may yield useful insights, the dissimilarities between the metaphor and its subject, if not acknowledged, can distort or pollute one's understanding of the subject. If attributes of the metaphor

are erroneously or misleadingly assigned to the subject and the distortion goes unchallenged, then the metaphor may alter the understanding of the underlying subject. The more appealing and powerful a metaphor, the more it tends to supplant or overshadow the original subject, and *the more one is unable to contemplate the subject apart from its metaphoric formulation*. Thus, distortions perpetuated by the metaphor are sustained and even magnified. This is the lesson of the "wall of separation" metaphor.[1]

And this, too, is the lesson of the "mental illness" metaphor.

Acknowledgments

THIS BOOK IS A SELECTION OF ESSAYS presented or published between 1972 and 2006. Grateful acknowledgment is made to the following sources for permission to use the articles that appear in this volume in adapted form:

1. "Mental Illness: A Metaphorical Disease." Adapted from "Mental Illness as a Metaphor," *Nature* 242 (March 30, 1973): 305–7. This article is a slightly modified and expanded version of my introductory remarks on the BBC television program *Controversy,* recorded at the Royal Institution on July 27, 1972, and broadcast on October 2, 1972. Reprinted without alteration, except for changing British to American spelling and omitting some references.

2. "Mental Illness: The New Phlogiston." Adapted from "Mental Illness: Psychiatry's Phlogiston," *Journal of Medical Ethics* 27 (October 2001): 297–301.

3. "Might Makes the Metaphor." Adapted from "Might Makes the Metaphor," *Journal of the American Medical Association* 229 (September 2, 1974): 1326. Copyright © 1974, American Medical Association. All rights reserved.

4. "Diagnosis: From Description to Prescription." Adapted from "Diagnosis in the Therapeutic State," *Liberty* 7 (September 1994): 25–28.

5. "Diagnoses Are Not Diseases." Adapted from "Diagnoses Are Not Diseases," *Lancet* 338 (December 21/28, 1991): 1574–76.

6. "The Existential Identity Thief." Adapted from "Bertrand Russell, C. S. Lewis, and the Existential Identity Thief," *Free Inquiry* 26 (August/September 2006): 51–52.

7. "Defining Disease." Adapted from "Defining Disease: The Gold Standard of Disease versus the Fiat Standard of Diagnosis." This chapter

appears with permission of the publisher from *The Independent Review: A Journal of Political Economy* 10 (Winter 2006): 325–36. © Copyright 2006, The Independent Institute, 100 Swan Way, Oakland, California 94621-1428; info@independent.org; www.independent.org.

8. "The Origin of Psychiatry: Coercion as Cure." Adapted from "The Origin of Psychiatry: The Alienist as Nanny for Troublesome Adults." *History of Psychiatry* 6 (1995): 1–19. Reprinted with permission of Sage Publications Ltd. Copyright © Sage Publications, 1995.

9. "Hysteria as Language." Adapted from: "Hysteria," In *International Encyclopedia of the Social Sciences,* ed. David L. Sills (New York: Macmillan & Free Press, 1968), 7: 47–52. Reprinted with permission of Gale, a division of Thomson Learning: www.thomsonrights.com. Fax 800 730-2215.

10. "Routine Neonatal Circumcision: A Medical Ritual." Adapted from an invited address delivered at the Third International Conference on Circumcision, Baltimore, Maryland, May 25, 1994. "Routine Neonatal Circumcision: Symbol of the Birth of the Therapeutic State," *Journal of Medicine and Philosophy* 21 (1996): 137–48. Reprinted with permission of Taylor and Francis.

11. "The Fatal Temptation: Drug Control and Suicide." Adapted from "The Fatal Temptation: Drug Prohibition and the Fear of Autonomy," *Daedalus* 121 (Summer 1992): 161–64.

12. "Pedophilia Therapy." Adapted from "Sins of the Fathers: Is Child Molestation a Sickness or a Crime?" *Reason* 34 (August 2002): 54–59.

13. "Psychiatry's War on Criminal Responsibility." Adapted from "The Psychiatrist in Court: People of the State of California v. Darlin June Cromer," *American Journal of Forensic Psychiatry* 3 (1982): 5–46; and "Reply to Simon," in *Szasz under Fire: The Psychiatric Abolitionist Faces His Critics,* ed. Jeffrey A. Schaler, (Chicago: Open Court, 2004), 202–23.

14. "Killing as Therapy: The Case of Terri Schiavo." Adapted from my keynote address, "Controversies in End of Life Care: Terri Schiavo's Lessons," Baystate Medical Center, Department of Psychiatry; Smith College School of Social Work; Baystate Health Systems, Office of Continuing Education. Smith College, Northampton, Massachusetts, October 10 and 11, 2005. "'A Rose for Emily,' a Rose for Terri: The Lifeless Body as Love Object and the Case of Theresa Marie Schindler Schiavo," *Palliative and*

Supportive Care 4 (June 2006): 159–67. Reprinted with permission of Cambridge University Press.

15. "Peter Singer's Ethics of Medicalization." Adapted from my contribution to the "Symposium: The Shifting Grounds of Life and Death," *Society* (July/August 2001). The symposium consisted of a lead essay by Peter Singer and six responses to it. Copyright © (2001) by Transaction Publishers. Reprinted by permission of the publisher.

16. "Pharmacracy: The New Despotism." Adapted from "The Therapeutic State: The Tyranny of Pharmacracy." This chapter appears with permission of the publisher from *The Independent Review: A Journal of Political Economy* 5 (Spring 2001): 485–521. © Copyright 2001, The Independent Institute, 100 Swan Way, Oakland, California 94621-1428; info@independent.org; www.independent.org.

I THANK MIRA DE VRIES for valuable suggestions, Roger Yanow for faithful help, and Sharon Givens for scanning essays written before I switched from typewriter to computer and for her generous secretarial help.

THOMAS SZASZ is professor emeritus of psychiatry at the State University of New York Upstate Medical University in Syracuse. The author of more than six hundred articles and thirty-two books, he is widely recognized as the leading critic of the coercive interventions employed by the psychiatric establishment.

Introduction

Woe unto you . . . for ye have taken away the key of knowledge.
—Luke 11:52

I

WHAT IS MEDICALIZATION? The *Merriam-Webster Online Dictionary* defines "medicalize" as "to view or treat as a medical concern, problem, or disorder" and offers this phrase as illustration: "those who seek to dispose of social problems by *medicalizing* them." Accordingly, we speak of the medicalization of homosexuality and racism, but do not speak of the medicalization of malaria or melanoma.

The concept of medicalization rests on the assumption that some phenomena belong in the domain of medicine, and some do not. Accordingly, unless we agree on *clearly defined* criteria that define membership in the class called "disease" or "medical problem," it is fruitless to debate whether any particular act of medicalization is "valid" or not.

Everything that we do or happens to us affects or depends on the use of our body. In principle, we could treat everything that people do or that happens to them as belonging in the domain of medicine. Conversely, we could maintain that nothing that we do or happens to us belongs in the domain of medicine because all is ordained by God and belongs in the domain of religion. Such, indeed, was the case in ancient times, before people distinguished between faith healing and medical healing. A similar view is held today by Christian Scientists, whose faith is based on a radical denial of the reality of the material world. For them, only the spiritual realm exists or is "real." Nothing belongs in the domain of materialist medicine. Christian Science represents the most radical case of demedicalization possible. Mary

Baker Eddy's foundational book, let us remember, was titled *Science and Health with Key to the Scriptures* (1875).

Contemporary public health may be regarded as the mirror image of Christian Science. Everything in our lives—housing, food, education, work, recreation, and procreation—affects our health. Therefore everything—not only health care narrowly defined—belongs in the domain of medicine as health care. Linda Landesman, a former president of the Public Health Association of New York City, states, "We expect and demand that government ensure that we breathe clean air, drink safe water, work with minimum danger, have medications where the benefits outweigh the risks and receive quality health care. . . . Left on our own, we don't always make the healthiest choices."[1] In this view, we are uninformed, undisciplined children whose health and well-being require the unremitting protection of the therapeutic state.

In practice, we must draw a line between what counts as medical care and what does not. The question is where to draw that line. What is a disease and what is not? What should be treated medically, by physicians or medical personnel, and what should not? Because people in modern societies expect the state to defray all or part of the cost of what is deemed a "medical service," where we draw the line between "health care" and "not health care" is informed more by economic and political considerations than by medical or scientific judgments.

Moreover, not only must we demarcate disease from nondisease, we must also distinguish between medicalization from above, by coercion, and medicalization from below, by choice. Not by coincidence, these *strategies* match psychiatry's two paradigmatic legal-social functions, civil commitment and the insanity defense, social control and excuse making.

II

The difference between disease as objective physical condition and the patient role as social status is obvious, provided we are willing to see it. Having a disease and occupying the patient role are independent variables: not all sick persons are patients, and not all patients are sick.[2] Physicians, politicians, the press, and the public nevertheless continue to confuse and conflate the two categories.³ This is a cultural setting conducive to the growth of medicalization. Oblivious of the distinction between diagnosis and disease and between disease and patient role, even critics who recognize that the American *furor diagnosticus* is spiraling out of control are helpless. For example, in a *Wall Street Journal* editorial in 1997, Jim Windolf, executive editor of the *New York Observer*, stated:

> The experts won't be satisfied until every last American is suffering from some kind of disease or disorder or syndrome. If you add together all the numbers compiled in the U.S. by all the institutes, the councils, the foundations, the Ph.D.'s and authors, you come up with one sorry statistical portrait of a nation. . . . With another new quantifiable disorder or two, everybody in America will be officially nuts.⁴

Being officially nuts is like being officially heretical or un-American, not like being infected with malaria. This point may be clarified by adding a few remarks about the opposite of medicalization, that is, demedicalization. Masturbation and homosexuality were, until relatively recently, considered diseases. Today, they no longer are. Have they been cured out of existence? No. They have been demedicalized. At the same time, hundreds of behaviors or habits never before treated as medical problems are now diagnosed as diseases: for example, drug abuse, social anxiety, and factitious disorder. Have these new diseases been discovered? No. They have been invented, that is, they are the products of medicalization. Moreover, these new diseases have been created pari passu with huge advances in the scientific detection of bodily diseases.

Ironically, technological advances in medicine, combined with the conflation of the concepts of disease and patient role, facilitate not only medicalization but also confusion between discovering diseases and creating diagnoses. As a result, when behaviors categorized as diseases are "declassified"—as happened with homosexuality—journalists, science writers, and the public are easily persuaded by the stakeholders in medicalization that demedicalization is also a product of scientific progress and moral enlightenment, and not the product of a power struggle between stigmatizers and stigmatized.

Medicalization is not a new phenomenon. (Neither is demedicalization, about which more in a moment.) Wherever diseased or disabled persons receive care or are excused from certain obligations, the condition is ripe for nondiseased and nondisabled individuals to pretend that they are sick or disabled. Formerly, people spoke about imaginary diseases and persons who pretended to be ill. Molière (1622–1673), the great satirist of malingerers and of the quacks whose harmful ministrations they invite, titled one his plays *The Imaginary Invalid (Le malade imaginaire)*. Among his memorable characters is Lucinde, a young bride in *The Doctor in Spite of Himself (Le médecin malgré lui),* who pretends to be unable to speak to avoid having to marry an old man her father wants her to wed ("hysterical aphonia").

Medicalization from below, from powerlessness—that is, malingering or self-medicalization—is an old phenomenon. Medicalization from above, from power—that is, medicalization of the other to control and punish—is a later development, associated with the birth of psychiatry. *Ward No. 6,* a gripping short story by Anton Chekhov (1860–1904), is an outstanding literary representation of psychiatry as medicalization from above. Andrew Efimich—the madhouse doctor who, in the end, is himself incarcerated as mad—addresses an inmate who begs to be freed:

> You ask me, what's to be done. The best thing to do in your situation is to escape from here. But, regrettably, that is useless. You would be detained. When society fences itself off from criminals, psychopaths, and people who are generally embarrassing, it is insuperable. There is but one thing left for you: to find reassurance in the thought that your staying here is necessary. . . . Since prisons and madhouses exist, why, somebody is bound to sit in them. If not you, then I. If not I, some third person. Bide your time: when in the distant future prisons and madhouses will have gone out of existence, there will be no more bars on windows nor hospital robes. Of course, sooner or later, such a time will come.[5]

A more recent literary example of medicalization as medical ideology, minus psychiatry, is a satirical play by Jules Romains (1885–1972), *Dr. Knock (Knock, ou le triomphe de médecine, 1923)*. Dr. Knock, the protagonist, declares:

Healthy people are sick people who don't know it. . . . "Get sick" is an old idea. It can't stand up to modern science. "Health" is a word we could just as well erase from our vocabularies. . . . It's a matter of principle with me to regard the entire population as our patients. Ipso facto. If you think it over, you'll be struck by its relation to the admirable concept of the nation in arms, a concept from which our modern states derive their strength.[6]

This image soon became stark reality in Germany, where physicians rushed to abandon the Hippocratic tradition and assume the roles of "biological soldiers" in the service of the *Vaterland*.[7]

III

How are we to understand medicalization and the confusion that reigns about what counts as a disease? Not by attributing it to scientific progress or cultural forces, as psychiatrists and psychiatric apologists are wont to do, but by identifying the medicalizers and exposing their motives. The view advanced by Charles E. Rosenberg, a distinguished professor of the history of science and the social sciences at Harvard University, is characteristically misleading:

Medicalization might perhaps be better understood as a long-term trend in Western society toward reductionist, somatic, and—increasingly—disease-specific explanations of human feelings and behavior *as well as unambiguously physical ills*. . . . Behavioral and emotional ills seem more accessible than "somatic" ills to lay people, who often question such categories as depression or attention deficit but rarely interrogate and are generally unaware of the indeterminacy built into the diagnosis or staging of a somatic ill such as cancer. . . . But the range of human dilemmas that we ask medicine to address has if anything expanded, from depression to anxiety, from bereavement to dysfunctional marriage. . . . So long as medicine in general and psychiatry in particular remains our designated manager of such problems, specific disease categories will always be an indispensable tool in the performance of that social role. . . . psychiatry and its concepts bleed constantly and unavoidably into the larger culture.[8]

Note that Rosenberg contrasts "human feelings and behavior" and "physical ills," and "behavioral ills" and "'somatic' ills," but does not tell us what his criteria are for distinguishing between them. Medicalization is not an impersonal process, as Rosenberg pretends. It is psychiatric propaganda, not historical analysis. In Rosenberg's account of medicalization, there are no agents, no winners or losers, and no one is responsible for the process: "psychiatry [that is, the manufacture of fictitious diseases] . . . bleeds into the larger culture." Bleeding may be started or stopped. Homosexuality became a mental illness when psychiatrists, wielding social power, claimed that it was; it became a nondisease when the homosexual lobby became powerful and troublesome enough to force psychiatrists to abolish the diagnosis.

The story of the medicalization and demedicalization of homosexuality highlights that medical classification—the linguistic-conceptual ordering of the phenomena we call "diseases" and of the interventions we call "treatments"—is a human activity, governed by human interests. In the United States today, the forces of medicalization rule virtually unopposed, indeed unrecognized for the economic, moral, and political interests that they represent. Our drug policies are illustrative. For millennia, the regulation of drug use was a matter of self-control, custom, religion, law. This is still, in part, the case. More importantly, however, drug use is regulated by ostensibly medical-scientific "facts" and medical-legal controls, exemplified by a broadly based drug prohibition consisting of prescription laws and the criminalization of trade in many drugs, such as heroin and marijuana. This is drug medicalization from above. Drug medicalization from below is pursued no less zealously by individuals who, while ostensibly opposed to our drug laws, promote so-called medical marijuana initiatives, physician-assisted suicide, and similar schemes. The result is loss of self-ownership and the right to self-medication—the classical liberal/libertarian perspective on drug use.

It would be difficult to exaggerate the importance of distinguishing between two kinds of patient roles: one forcibly ascribed, another voluntarily assumed. In psychiatry, the patient role is typically ascribed to persons diagnosed as psychotic or schizophrenic, and is typically assumed by persons diagnosed as suffering from hypochondriasis, hysteria, conversion reaction, somatization, factitious illness, and so forth.

IV

In his influential book *The Concept of Mind,* Oxford philosopher Gilbert Ryle introduced the concept of "category error."[9] Ryle's thesis was simple, indeed elementary: the predication of substance is not meaningful for a disposition or capacity. Therefore, it is a mistake to treat the mind as an object. Because the mind is not an object, like the body, it is a mistake to apply the predicate *disease* to it. The "diseased mind" is a metaphor, a mistake, a myth.[10]

This is not a new idea. Emil Kraepelin (1856–1927), the creator of the first modern psychiatric nosology, acknowledged the fundamental analytic truth that there are no mental illnesses. In his classic, *Lectures on Clinical Psychiatry* (1901), he stated, "The subject of the following course of lectures will be the Science of Psychiatry, which, as its name [*Seelenheilkunde*] implies, is that of the treatment of mental disease. *It is true that, in the strictest terms, we cannot speak of the mind as becoming diseased [Allerdings kann mann, streng genommen, nicht von Erkrankungen der Seele sprechen].*"[11] Half a century earlier, the Viennese psychiatrist Ernst von Feuchtersleben (1806–1848) explicitly emphasized the analogical-metaphorical character of mental illnesses: "The maladies of the spirit [*die Leiden des Geistes*] alone, *in abstracto,* that is, error and sin, can be called diseases of the mind only *per analogiam.* They come not within the jurisdiction of the physician, but that of the teacher or clergyman, who again are called *physicians of the mind [Seelenärzte]* only *per analogiam.*"[12]

However, Ryle's concept of category error is grievously incomplete. It ignores that treating the mind—mental symptom, mental illness, psychopathology, the unconscious—as an object may be a strategy, not an error or mistake; that the "error" is not innocent; that, depending on circumstances, it benefits some and harms others; that, today, there is fame, money, power, and escape from responsibility in the medicalization of everyday life, obloquy, marginalization, and worse in opposition to it.

The transformation of religious explanations and controls into medical explanations and controls of behavior is one of the momentous consequences of the Enlightenment. The waning power of religion and the Church and the waxing power of science and the nation state is manifested, among other things, by the political control of medical practice and the drug laws that deny access to lay person to drugs (except those classified as over the counter). To legally obtain or possess a "prescription drug," the lay person must establish a professional relationship with a licensed physician and receive a diagnosis for an illness: that is, he must be a patient who suffers from a proven or putative illness. For example, to receive a sleeping pill, the person must "suffer from insomnia." This charade contributes mightily to the medicalization rampant in our society. In turn, medicalization is mindlessly equated, especially by the cognoscenti, with scientific, moral, and social progress, and contributes further to its popularity.

V

Although medicalization encompasses more than psychiatry, we must be clear about one thing: *Psychiatry is medicalization, through and through.* Whatever aspect of psychiatry psychiatrists claim is not medicalization, is not medicalization only if it deals with proven disease, in which case it belongs to neurology, neuroanatomy, neurophysiology, neurochemistry, neuropharmacology, or neurosurgery, not psychiatry.

Psychoanalysis is medicalization squared. It is important, in this connection, not to be fooled by lay analysis, clinical psychology, or social work. These and other nonmedical mental health and counseling "professions" are medicalization cubed: as if to compensate for their lack of medical qualifications, nonmedical mental health "professionals" are even more deeply committed than psychiatrists to their claim of special expertise in the diagnosis and treatment of mental illnesses.[13]

By the time Sigmund Freud (1856–1939) appeared on the historical stage, medicalization was in full swing. The birth of psychoanalysis is, in fact, a manifestation of the increasing popularity of this trend at the end of the nineteenth century as well as a cause of its explosive growth during the twentieth century. In 1901 Freud published one of his favorite works, revealingly titled *The Psychopathology of Everyday Life*.[14] The gist of Freud's thesis was that the symptoms of mental illnesses are the "products" of the same "mental processes" that are responsible for the thoughts and actions of normal persons. In other words, Freud rediscovered that "there is method in madness," or, as he preferred to put it, that sane and insane behaviors are subject to the same "psychological laws." To create his special brand of pseudoscience, he titled his book *The Psychopathology of Everyday Life*. He could just as well have titled it *The Everyday Normality of the Psychopathological Life*. There would, of course, have been neither fame nor fortune in that. Instead, he chose to enflame medicalization and managed to transform a smoldering fire into an all-consuming conflagration. At the same time, because Freud knew better, his attitude toward medicalization throughout his long life was ambivalent and opportunistic. Most of the time, he was an enthusiastic medicalizer:

The neuroses are a particular kind of illness and analysis is a particular method of treating them, a specialized branch of medicine.[15]

The first piece of reality with which the patient must deal is his illness[16]

[T]hey [the neuroses] are severe, constitutionally fixed illnesses, which rarely restrict themselves to only a few attacks but persist as a rule over long periods or throughout life.[17]

I was thus led into regarding the neuroses as being without exception disturbances of the sexual function. . . . My medical conscience felt pleased at my having arrived at this conclusion[18]

Psychoanalysis is really a method of treatment like others.[19]

At other times, when it suited his purpose, Freud resisted the medicalization of psychoanalysis:

I have assumed, that is to say, that psychoanalysis is not a specialized branch of medicine. I cannot see how it is possible to dispute this.[20]

[I]n his medical school a doctor receives a training which is more or less the opposite of what he would need as a preparation for psychoanalysis.[21]

It may perhaps turn out that in this instance the patients are not like other patients . . . [22]

We [analysts] serve the patient . . . as a teacher and educator.[23]

Furthermore, it is in *The Psychopathology of Everyday Life* that Freud first lays claim to the mantle of scientist: "If the distinction between conscious and unconscious motivation is taken into account, our feeling of conviction informs us that conscious motivation does not extend to all our motor decisions. . . . what is thus left free by the one side receives its motivation from the other side, from the unconscious; and in this way determination in the psychical sphere is still carried out without any gap."[24]

Freud believed that his allegiance to "scientific determinism" and denial of free will were evidence of his scientific bona fides. In fact, they reveal the conventionality of his cast of mind. In large part, Freud labored in the same vineyard of sexual medicalization that his colleague Baron Richard von Krafft-Ebing (1840–1902) had staked out. He extended Krafft-Ebing's psychopathologizing of behavior from sexual life to everyday life, inverting Shakespeare's proto-existential interpretations of human conflict into dehumanized interpretations of tragedy as symptoms of psychopathology.[25]

Krafft-Ebing, a German-born professor of psychiatry at the University of Vienna, was a world-famous figure, largely because of the sensation caused by his book *Psychopathia Sexualis* (1886). Thanks to his pioneering efforts, sexual desires and aversions in their manifold forms became an integral part of medicine and the new science of psychiatry. To impress the medical character of his work on the profession and the public, Krafft-Ebing sprinkled his text liberally with Latin, and he and his publisher alike maintained that *Psychopathia Sexualis* was written only for medical professionals, solely for medical use. In the preface to the first edition, Krafft-Ebing wrote, "The object of this treatise is merely to record the various *psychopathological manifestations of sexual life in man*. . . . The physician finds, perhaps, a solace in the fact that he may at times refer those manifestations which offend against our ethical and aesthetical principles to a diseased condition of the mind or the body."[26] I list, without further comment, some of the "diseases" Krafft-Ebing identified as "Cerebral Neuroses": "*Anaesthesia* (absence of sexual instinct) . . . *Hyperaesthesia* (increased desire, satyriasis) . . . *Paraesthesia* (perversion of the sexual instinct) . . . *Fetishism* invests imaginary presentations of separate parts of the body or portions of raiment of the opposite sex . . . with voluptuous sensations."[27]

The public's memory is short. Towards the end of nineteenth century, doctors transformed diverse human sexual appetites and practices into a Latin dictionary of diseases. A hundred years later, they transformed many of those diseases—for example, masturbation, pornography, and prostitution—into "sex therapy."[28] The new quacks—led by William Masters and Virginia Johnson—became celebrated "doctors" and "scientists." Their best-selling sex manuals were full of gems of medicalization such as this one: "a physician, frankly quite curious about the partner-surrogate role, offered her services to evaluate the potentials (if any) of the role. When convinced of the desperate need for such a partner in the treatment of sexual dysfunction in the unmarried male, she continued as a partner surrogate, contributing both personal and professional experiences to develop the role to a peak of effectiveness. The therapists [that is, Masters and Johnson] are indeed more than indebted to this intelligent woman."[29] This is medicalization running amok. Note that Masters and Johnson speak of being indebted to "this woman." They do not call her "doctor," or "physician," or "prostitute," and do not tell us whether or how much she charged for her sex therapy sessions.

VI

People do not have to be told that malaria and melanoma are diseases. They know they are. But people have to be told, and are told over and over again, that alcoholism and depression are diseases. Why? Because people know that they are not diseases: that mental illnesses are not "like other illnesses," that mental hospitals are not like other hospitals, that the business of psychiatry is coercion, not cure.[30] Accordingly, medicalizers engage in a never-ending task of "educating" people that nondiseases are diseases. Herewith some examples.

The Johnson Institute, founded by Dr. Vernon Johnson, an Episcopal priest and self-styled "recovered alcoholic," is one of the major American antialcoholism organizations. The institute's aim is to medicalize the (excessive) drinking of alcoholic beverages. At a forum held at the National Press Club in Washington, D.C., in 2004, attended by "more than 50 leaders representing 85 organizations," Dr. David C. Lewis, founder of the Center for Alcoholism and Addiction Studies at Brown University, explained:

"Addiction treatment needs to be considered a more mainstream medical procedure such as treatments for cancer, depression and other chronic diseases." Dr. Ron Hunsicker, president and CEO of the National Association of Addiction Treatment Providers, warned, "[T]he focus must be to keep addictions as a public health issue and not a social services issue. We must resist every attempt to have alcoholism and drug addiction seen as anything but a medical issue. . . . It's a primary disease, not symptomatic of some other disease."[31]

The medicalizers of depression are equally numerous and aggressive. One group of depression medicalizers, the "Depression Is Real Coalition," is supported by the American Psychiatric Foundation, Depression and Bipolar Support Alliance, League of United Latin American Citizens, National Alliance on Mental Illness, National Medical Association, National Mental Health Association, and the National Urban League. The coalition's Web site states that it is "a group of seven nonprofit organizations representing doctors, people living with mental illness and American communities. . . . We have come together to help educate the public about the true nature of depression and to offer hope."[32]

During October 2006, under the photo of Dr. Paul Greengard, 2000 Nobel laureate in medicine, endorsing its message, the coalition published full-page ads in magazines that stated:

> Every year, without any treatment at all, thousands stop suffering from depression. Because it kills them. . . . We want people to realize that depression is a real and very serious medical illness with a biological basis. If you or someone you care about has ever suffered from depression, you know Depression Is Real. But if you watch TV, read the popular press or search the Internet, you will find all kinds of confusing messages. You may have heard that depression is "just the blues" or worse a "made-up disease." Those kinds of statements obscure the real facts about a debilitating and potentially deadly medical condition that affects some 19 million Americans every year. So, while Depression Is Real, hope is real, too.[33]

Formerly, people *felt* depressed or *were* depressed. Now they *have* depression. Formerly, some depressed persons killed themselves, but most did not. Now people do not kill themselves, *depression kills them,* and (virtually) all who kill themselves are said to have been depressed. And just as people can have cancer and not know it, so they may have depression and not know it, and hence need to be tested for it, lest "it" kill them. On its Web site, the Depression Is Real Coalition emphasizes:

> *Indisputable scientific evidence shows depression to be a biologically-based disease that destroys the connections between brain cells* . . . The Depression Is Real campaign consists of television, radio and print public service announcements (PSAs), print and radio advertisements, a Web site (www. DepressionIsReal.org), and other educational activities. The print and radio ads are science-based and feature Dr. Paul Greengard, winner of the 2000 Nobel Prize in Physiology/Medicine and an expert in brain function and the mechanisms of depression. . . . The Depression Is Real Coalition is particularly concerned that depression is not widely recognized or taken seriously enough in the African-American and Latino communities, which are already underserved in many areas of health care.[34]

At the same time, the National Mental Health Association launched a campaign aimed especially at the college student population, titled "Finding Hope and Help: College Student and Depression Pilot Initiative":

> Depression affects over 19 million American adults annually, including college students. At colleges nationwide, large percentages of college students are feeling overwhelmed, sad, hopeless and so depressed that they are unable to function. According to a recent national college health survey, 10% of college students have been diagnosed with depression. . . . Women are five times as likely to have anxiety disorders. Eating disorders affect 5–10 million women and 1 million men, with the highest rates occurring in college-aged women. Suicide was the eighth leading cause of death for all Americans, the third leading cause of death for those aged 15–24, and the second leading killer in the college population in 1998. . . . More than 30% of college freshmen report feeling overwhelmed a great deal of the time. About 38% of college women report feeling frequently overwhelmed. . . . For more information about the National Mental Health Association's (NMHA) College Student and Depression Initiative, contact: College Student and Depression Initiative . . . *The Initiative is made possible through educational grants from AstraZeneca, Bristol-Myers Squibb Company, The*

E.H.A. Foundation, Eli Lilly and Company, Forest Laboratories, Inc., Glaxo-SmithKline, Pfizer Inc, and Wyeth.[35]

Cui bono? The answer is obvious. It is also obvious that the self-styled psychiatric "educators" never mention two major risks inherent in every professional contact between an individual and a psychiatrist, namely, stigmatization by diagnosis and loss of liberty by forced psychiatric "hospitalization." Why do the promoters of medicalization—that is, psychiatric slavery—regularly fail to mention its potential downside? Because they mendaciously regard psychiatric oppression of the patient as beneficial for that patient, much as the promoters of chattel slavery regarded oppression of slaves as beneficial for them. Lincoln's answer to this outrage remains relevant: "But, slavery is good for some people! As a good thing, slavery is strikingly peculiar, in this, that it is the only good thing which no man ever seeks the good of, for himself."[36]

In short, medicalization is not medicine or science; it is a semantic-social strategy that benefits some persons and harms others.

Egas Moniz, a Nobel laureate in medicine, lent his name and prestige to the worldwide iatrogenic plague of curing nondiseases by lobotomy, typically imposed on the subject against his will or without his consent. Sadly, now another Nobel laureate in medicine, Paul Greengard, lends his name and prestige to a new worldwide iatrogenic plague of curing nondisease by chemotherapy, fraudulently or forcibly imposed on the subject. Any psychiatric campaign that deserves the name "education" ought to begin by emphasizing these risks.

"[T]he medical treatment of [mental] patients began with the infringement of their personal freedom,"[37] warned Karl Wernicke (1848–1905), the pioneer German neuropathologist. It still begins with the infringement of their personal freedom.

PART ONE

Demarcating Disease from Nondisease

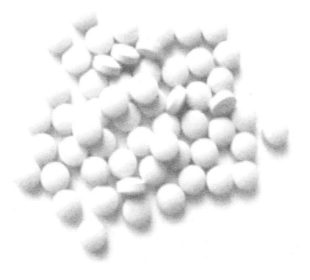

1

Mental Illness

A Metaphorical Disease

Metaphor: a figure of speech in which a word or phrase literally denoting
one kind of object or idea is used in place of another to suggest a likeness
or analogy between them (as in *drowning in money*).
                    —*Merriam-Webster Online Dictionary*

I

ABOUT TWENTY YEARS AGO (that is, in the early 1950s) I began to
clarify what seemed to me the core problem of psychiatry—namely, the nature of so-called mental illness. This led to a systematic scrutiny and refu-
tation of the two fundamental claims of contemporary psychiatrists—that
mental illnesses are genuine diseases, and that psychiatry is a bona fide
medical specialty.[1]

It is impossible to undertake an analysis of the concept of mental illness
without first coming to grips with the concept of ordinary or bodily illness.
What do we mean when we say that a person is ill? We usually mean two
quite different things: first, that he believes, or that his physician believes, or
that they both believe, that he suffers from an abnormality or malfunction-
ing of his body; and second, that he wants, or is at least willing to accept,
medical help for his suffering. The term "illness" thus refers, first, to an abnormal biological condition whose existence may be claimed, truly or falsely,
by patient, physician, or others; and second, to the social role of the patient,
which may be assumed or assigned.

If a person does not suffer from an abnormal biological condition, we do
not usually consider him to be ill. (We certainly do not consider him to be

physically ill.) And if he does not voluntarily assume the role of one who is sick, he is not usually considered to be a medical patient. This is because the practice of modern Western medicine rests on two tacit premises—namely, that the physician's task is to diagnose and treat disorders of the human body and that he can carry out these services only with the consent of his patient. In other words, physicians are trained to treat bodily ills—not economic, moral, racial, religious, or political "ills." And they themselves (except psychiatrists) expect, and in turn are expected by their patients, to treat bodily diseases, not envy and rage, fear and folly, poverty and stupidity, and all the other miseries that beset man. Strictly speaking, then, disease or illness can affect only the body. Hence, there can be no such thing as mental illness. The term "mental illness" is a metaphor.

II

To understand current psychiatric practices, it is necessary to understand how and why the idea of mental illness arose and the way it now functions. In part, the concept of mental illness arose from the fact that it is possible for a person to act and to appear as if he were sick without actually having a bodily disease. How should we react to such a person? Should we treat him as if he were not ill or as if he were ill?

Until the second half of the nineteenth century, persons who imitated illness—that is, who claimed to be sick without being able to convince their physicians that they suffered from bona fide illnesses—were regarded as faking illness and were called malingerers; and those who imitated medical practitioners—that is, who claimed to heal the sick without being able to convince medical authorities that they were bona fide physicians—were regarded as impostors and were called quacks.

As a result of the influence of Charcot, Janet, and especially Freud, the perspective, both medical and lay, on imitations of illness and healing was radically transformed. Henceforth, persons who imitated illness—for example, who had "spells"—were regarded as genuinely ill and were called hysterics; and those who imitated physicians—for example, who "hypnotized"—were regarded as genuine healers and were called psychotherapists. This profound conceptual transformation was both supported and reflected by an equally profound semantic transformation—one in which "spells," for example, became "seizures" and "quacks" became "psychoanalysts."

A few brief quotations from Freud's early writings must suffice to support my contentions. In 1893, Freud wrote that "hysteria has fairly often been credited with a faculty for simulating the most various organic nervous disorders."[2] While seeming to offer a simple description of the characteristics of the disease called "hysteria," Freud here falsifies the historical record.

Most of the contemporaries and predecessors of the young Freud credited not hysteria but malingerers with the "faculty for simulating." Indeed, being an abstraction and a name, hysteria cannot simulate or imitate anything; only persons can. Nor is this an isolated figure of speech or stylistic peculiarity of Freud's; on the contrary, it is a part of his systematic strategy for reifying and personalizing pseudomedical labels and for stigmatizing and depersonalizing persons. Thus, in the same paper, Freud asserts that "hysteria behaves as though anatomy did not exist or as though it had no knowledge of it."[3] But hysteria neither behaves nor knows; only persons do.

In the same year, Breuer and Freud made their now famous announcement that "hysterics suffer mainly from reminiscences."[4] Here we are offered a metaphorical expression as if it were a literal one: for in the context in which it occurs, the statement implies that hysterics suffer from reminiscences in the same way as arteriosclerotics suffer from hardening of the arteries. But reminiscences are not real lesions; nor, therefore, are hysterics real patients.

Lastly, in a paper published in 1909, Freud acknowledges that the hysteric fakes illness. By then hysteria was well enough established as a legitimate illness, and Freud did not use such direct language to say so. What he said was that "[hysterical] attacks are nothing else but phantasies translated into the motor sphere, projected on to motility and portrayed in pantomime."[5] In plain English: hysteria is the dramatic imitation of illness. Nevertheless, Freud would have us believe that hysteria is itself an illness.

The upshot of this psychiatric-psychoanalytic "revolution" is that, today, it is considered shamefully uncivilized and naively unscientific to treat a person who acts or appears sick as if he were not sick. We now "know" and "realize" that such a person is sick; that he is obviously sick; that he is mentally sick.

But this view rests on a serious, albeit simple, error: it rests on mistaking or confusing what is real with what is imitation, literal meaning with metaphorical meaning, medicine with morals. In other words, I maintain that mental illness is a metaphorical disease: that bodily illness stands in the same relation to mental illness as a defective television set stands to a bad television program. Of course, the word "sick" is often used metaphorically. We call jokes "sick," economies "sick," sometimes even the whole world "sick"; but only when we call minds "sick" do we systematically mistake and strategically misinterpret metaphor for fact—and send for the doctor to "cure" the "illness." It is as if a television viewer were to send for a television engineer because he dislikes the program he sees on the screen.

III

Such considerations lead to two diametrically opposed points of view about mental illness and psychiatry. According to the traditional and at present generally accepted view, mental illness is like any other illness, psychiatric treatment is like any other treatment, and psychiatry is like any other medical specialty. According to the view I have endeavored to develop and clarify, however, there is, and can be, no such thing as mental illness or psychiatric treatment; the interventions now designated as "psychiatric treatment" must be clearly identified as voluntary or involuntary: voluntary interventions are things a person does for himself in an effort to change, whereas involuntary interventions are things done to him in an effort to change him against his will; and psychiatry is not a medical but a moral and political enterprise.

Whereas illness is something a patient has or claims to have or is said to have, treatment is something a physician does or claims to do. Clearly, however, not everything a physician does constitutes treatment but only those of his interventions that are believed to be helpful or effective against the illness from which the patient suffers, and, among these, only those interventions to which the patient, assuming him to be a conscious adult, consents. In a free society, the fact that a person has an illness or that an illness is attributed to him—regardless of whether the illness is bodily or mental, literal or metaphorical—does not, and cannot, by itself justify imposing medical treatment on him against his will.

Thus, the quarantining of patients with certain contagious diseases has been justified, and can be justified, only by society's right to protect itself from the patient's illness; it cannot be justified by society's right to protect the patient from the consequences of his illness.

It is sometimes claimed that, like patients with contagious diseases, some patients with so-called mental diseases also "endanger society." The precise meaning and the factual validity of this claim are doubtful at best, and the use to which it is put—to justify the necessity of involuntary psychiatric interventions—is illogical and immoral. For if and when "mental patients" endanger or injure others, they do so not through their "illness" but through their behavior. That this is so is self-evident: it is inherent in our very ideas of contagious and mental diseases. Contagious diseases, such as syphilis or tuberculosis, are things that not only patients can have, but also corpses; whereas mental diseases, such as depression or psychopathy, are things that corpses assuredly can never have. Therefore, if and insofar as it is deemed that "mental patients" endanger society, society can, and ought to, protect itself from the "mentally ill" in the same way as it does from the "mentally healthy"—that is, by means of the criminal law. To be sure, society cannot do so as long as it recognizes "mental illness" as both an incriminating condition (as in involuntary hospitalization) and an excusing condition (as in the insanity defense and verdict).

In short, one of the fundamental moral and political implications of the views I have presented here is that one of our most important and most precious rights, and at present one of the most threatened, is the right to be ill— that is, the right to reject treatment, the right to suffer, and the right to die unmolested by interventions imposed upon us by the state acting through its medical (or psychiatric) agencies. In a theological society, we could not sin or die without the cleric, whether we wanted him or not. Mutatis mutandis, in a therapeutic society such as ours, we cannot be sick or die without the clinician, whether we want him or not.[6]

IV

Lest it be thought that these considerations apply only to psychiatric conditions and practices in the United States, I should like to conclude by calling attention to several recent cases reported in the British press.

First, there are the three women who had been incarcerated in psychiatric institutions for fifty years because of illegitimate pregnancies.[7] Perhaps it will be objected that that was long ago, and that such things no longer happen today. Of course not. Today women are hospitalized involuntarily not for having illegitimate babies but for having illegitimate ideas, which we conveniently call "delusions."

Second, there is the Jordanian eye doctor, the son of the Grand Mufti of Jerusalem, accused of killing three children, who was promptly found "unfit to plead," and was "detained in a hospital."[8]

And third, there is the case of Graham Young, tried only a few months ago, who, having been "cured" at Broadmoor of the disease of enjoying poisoning people, had an unfortunate relapse and poisoned several more.[9] Revealingly, his last bout of evil, though phenomenologically undistinguishable from his previous one, was not attributed to mental disease: this time he was sent to prison, not to Broadmoor. It is difficult to imagine a more clear-cut illustration of one of my basic propositions, namely, that what we call mental illness (especially in a legal context) is not a condition but a policy; not a fact but a strategy; in short, not a disease that the alleged patient has but a decision we make about how to act toward him, whether he likes it or not. I submit that each of these cases demonstrates an insistent denial of the differences between disease and deviance, between healing for the benefit of the suffering patient and social control for the protection of society, and between medical institutions whose clients are at liberty, because they are free adults, to leave the premises should they be dissatisfied with the service, and penal institutions whose inmates, because they are convicted offenders, are deliberately and explicitly deprived of this option.

What, then, is to be done? A few simple things; however, because of our intense devotion to the medical perspective on human problems, these may prove to be quite unpalatable.

First, as so-called mental health problems are not medical but human (that is, moral, social, and political) problems, we cannot solve them by therapeutic means; we must stop continuing and even intensifying our efforts to solve them by such means.

Second, since the vocabulary of psychiatry serves to systematically redefine moral and political problems as diseases, we must repudiate and stop this abuse of our language.

Third, as psychiatric "treatments" are chiefly overtly or covertly involuntary, such interventions must be disavowed; we must reject the use of psychiatrists as policemen, judges, and jailers; and we must seriously dedicate ourselves to the proposition that "mental health" workers should help only those who want to be helped, that they should do so only in ways acceptable to their clients, and that they should stop doing everything else.

2

Mental Illness

The New Phlogiston

There is no error so monstrous that it fails to find defenders among the ablest men.

—Lord Acton (1834–1902), "Democracy"

I

PEOPLE CRAVE ANSWERS, and the more ignorant and puzzled they are, the more numerous and confident are their answers. In a manner of speaking, therefore, everyone may be considered a would-be scientist. The true scientist differs from the ordinary person only in the depth, breadth, precision, and power of the account he accepts as the correct explanation for his observation, and in his willingness to revise it in the light of new evidence. In this essay, I will show that mental illness is to psychiatry as phlogiston was to chemistry.

In physics, we use the same laws to explain why airplanes fly and why they crash. In psychiatry, we use one set of laws to explain sane behavior, which we attribute to reasons (choices), and another set of laws to explain insane behavior, which we attribute to causes (diseases). God, man's idea of moral perfection, judges human deeds without distinguishing between sane persons responsible for their behavior and insane person deserving to be excused for their evil deeds. It is hubris to pretend that the insanity defense is compassionate, just, or scientific. Mental illness is to psychiatry as phlogiston was to chemistry. Establishing chemistry as a science of the nature of matter required the recognition of the nonexistence of phlogiston. Establishing psychiatry as a science of human behavior requires the recognition of the nonexistence of mental illness.

Chemistry began as alchemy, which, in turn, was closely connected with medicine. Both Johann Joachim Becher (1635–1682) and Georg Ernst Stahl (1660–1734), two of chemistry's pioneers, were physicians at a time when people believed that problems of health and disease are best explained in terms of the four basic Galenic humors.

One of foremost problems early chemists tried to solve was combustion. What happens when a substance burns? Stahl proposed that all flammable objects contained a material substance that he called "phlogiston," from the Greek word meaning "to set on fire." When a substance burned, it liberated its content of phlogiston into the air, which was believed to be chemically inert. The phlogiston theory dominated scientific thinking for more than a century.

However, it was observed that after a piece of metal was burned (oxidized) it weighed more than it did before, whereas according to the phlogiston theory it should have weighed less. This inconsistency was resolved by postulating that phlogiston was an immaterial principle rather than a material substance; alternatively, it was suggested that phlogiston had a negative weight. When chemists discovered hydrogen, they believed it to be pure phlogiston.

The phlogiston theory was overthrown by the work of Antoine Laurent Lavoisier (1743–1794). He named the fraction of air that supported combustion "oxygen," a term derived from the Greek words meaning "acid producing" because he thought, wrongly, that oxygen was a necessary component of all acids. The major fraction of air that does not support combustion he called "azote," from the Greek words meaning "no life." Azote is now called "nitrogen." In a historic paper, titled "Memoir on the Nature of the Principle which Combines with Metals during Their Calcination [oxidation] and which Increases Their Weight," delivered at the French Royal Academy of Sciences in 1775 and published in 1778, Lavoisier disproved the phlogiston theory and laid the framework for understanding chemical reactions as combinations of elements that form new materials.[1]

Once names and theories gain wide acceptance, they exercise a powerful influence on those inculcated to believe that their existence forms an integral part of the way the world is—in short, "reality." New observations are then "seen" through the lens of the prevailing system of mental optics.

For example, Joseph Priestley (1733-1804), the great English chemist, could not relinquish the phlogiston theory, even after he himself had discovered oxygen and after Lavoisier's work swept the scientific world. He continued to view oxygen as "dephlogisticated air." In a pamphlet titled "Considerations on the Doctrine of Phlogiston and the Decomposition of Water," published in 1796, he referred to Lavoisier's followers as "Antiphlogistians" and complained, "On the whole, I cannot help saying, that it appears to me not a little extraordinary, that a theory so new, and of such importance, overturning every thing that was thought to be the best established chemistry, should rest on so very narrow and precarious a foundation."[2]

While alchemy changed into chemistry, the soul changed into the mind and sin became sickness (of the mind). The early alienists frankly acknowledged this metamorphosis. However, instead of recognizing that it was an early manifestation of a move from a religious to a secular outlook on human behavior, they attributed it to scientific advances and believed to have discovered a set of new brain diseases and called them "mental diseases." What Georg Ernst Stahl was to early chemistry and phlogiston, Benjamin Rush (1745–1813) was to early psychiatry and mental illness.

II

Modern natural science rests on laws uninfluenced by human desire or motivation. We use the same physical laws to explain why airplanes fly and crash, the same chemical laws to explain the therapeutic and toxic effects of drugs, and the same biological laws to explain how healthy cells maintain the integrity of the organism and these cells can become cancerous and destroy the host. We do not have one set of medical theories to explain normal bodily functions, and another set to explain abnormal bodily functions.

In psychiatry, the situation is the reverse. We have one set of principles to explain the functioning of the mentally healthy person and another set to explain the functioning of the mentally ill person: we attribute acceptable, "rational" behaviors to *reasons,* unacceptable, "irrational" behaviors to *causes.* The mentally healthy person is viewed as an active agent. He makes decisions: he chooses, for example, to marry his sweetheart. In contrast, the mentally ill person is viewed as a passive body: as patient, he is the victim of injurious biological, chemical, or physical processes acting upon his body, that is, diseases (of his brain), for example, of an "irresistible impulse" to kill. "The epileptic neurosis," wrote Sir Henry Maudsley (1835–1918), the founder of modern British psychiatry, "is that it is apt to burst out into a convulsive explosion of violence. . . . To hold an insane person responsible for not controlling an insane impulse . . . is in some cases just as false . . . as it would be to hold a man convulsed by strychnia responsible for not stopping the convulsions."[3] It is a false analogy. Killing is a coordinated *act*. Convulsion is an uncoordinated contraction of muscles, an *event*.

Because explanations of human behavior influence law and social policy much more pervasively and profoundly than do explanations of natural events, the mental illness theory of behavior has far-reaching implications for virtually every aspect of our daily life. Law professor Michael S. Moore expresses a view now widely shared by lawyers, psychiatrists, and the general public:

> Since mental illness negates our assumption of rationality, we do not hold the mentally ill responsible. It is not so much that we excuse them from a prima facie case of responsibility; rather, by being unable to regard them as fully rational beings, we cannot affirm the essential condition to viewing them as moral agents to begin with. In this the mentally ill join (to a decreasing degree) infants, wild beasts, plants, and stones—none of which are responsible because of the absence of any assumption of rationality.[4]

We are proud that we have all but abolished our prejudiced beliefs about the differences between the human natures of men and women or whites and blacks. At the same time, we are even prouder that we have created a set of psychiatric beliefs about the differences between the neuroanatomical and neurophysiological natures of the sane and the insane, the mentally healthy and the mentally ill. Oxidation, a real process, explains combustion better than does phlogiston, a nonexistent substance. Attributing *all human actions* to choice, the basic building block of our social existence, explains human behavior better than attributing certain (disapproved) actions to mental illness, a nonexistent disease.

A cause may operate momentarily or over time. A stationary billiard ball begins to move the moment another ball hits it. A broken hip makes walking impossible for days or weeks. Therefore, it is not enough to say that a person pushes another in front of a subway train because he has schizophrenia and that schizophrenia is due to abnormal neurochemical processes in the brain. We must also explain why he did so when he did so. The alleged condition, "schizophrenia," cannot do that, inasmuch as it existed before the commission of the homicide and is said to exist in millions of persons who engage in no violence.

A person opens his umbrella when he goes out into the rain because he does not want to get wet. A person pushes another in front of a subway train not because he "has" schizophrenia or because schizophrenia "makes" him do it; he does it because, like the man who opens an umbrella, he wants to improve his existence. We can explain a person's seemingly irrational act too by attributing it to a reason, for example, wanting to attract attention to himself or wanting to escape responsibility for housing and feeding himself.

In short, regardless of the condition of an "irrationally" acting person's brain, he remains a moral agent who has reasons for his actions: like all of us, he chooses or wills what he does. People with brain diseases—amyotrophic lateral sclerosis, multiple sclerosis, Parkinsonism, glioblastoma—are persons whose actions continue to be governed by their desires or motives. The illness limits their freedom of action but not their status as moral agents.

III

According to psychiatric theory, certain actions by certain people ought to be attributed to causes, not reasons. When and why do we seek a causal explanation for personal conduct? When we consider the actor's behavior unreasonable and do not want to blame him for it. We then look for an excuse masquerading as an explanation, rather than simply an explanation that neither exonerates nor incriminates.

There is a crucial difference between explaining the movement of objects and explaining the behavior of persons. Our explanation of the movement of planets is (today) devoid of moral implications, whereas our explanation of the behavior of persons is heavily freighted with moral implications. As a rule, we hold persons responsible for what they do, and do not hold them responsible for what happens to them. Agreement and disagreement, approval and disapproval, praise and blame are tacit elements of the vocabulary we use to explain personal conduct.

Holding a person responsible for his act is not the same as blaming or praising him for it: it means only that we regard him as an actor or moral agent. Blame or praise expresses judgment of his act, or of him as a person, as wicked or virtuous; in either case, it does not gainsay his authorship of his behavior. Conversely, holding a person not responsible for his act by reason of mental illness means that we do not regard him as a (full-fledged) actor or moral agent; instead, we regard him as a victim of his "illness." Although we pronounce such a person "not guilty" of the injurious act he has committed (say, murder), we nevertheless regard his act as deplorable, and we nevertheless deprive him of liberty. We have not proved that he lacks reasons for his behavior. We have merely offered a different explanation for his behavior (based on causes, not reasons) and provided a different justification for detaining him (based on medical rather than legal considerations). In short, the insanity plea, insanity verdict, and insanity disposition form a tactical package we use if we do not want to regard an actor as a moral agent and prefer to "treat" him as a mental patient.

It is a mistake to believe that offering an excuse explanation for an act is tantamount to showing that the actor has no reasons for his action. Offering an excuse for doing X—"God's voice commanded me"—is not the same as not having reasons for doing X. To the contrary: what we have shown is not that the actor has no reasons but that his reasons are wrongheaded—"deluded," "mad," "insane." We conclude that his actions are *caused* by his being deluded, mad, insane. But we have not proven anything of the sort; we have postulated it.

Prior to the eighteenth century, people who committed heinous crimes and acted strangely were thought to resemble wild animals, hence, the antiquated "wild beast" model of insanity and the defense based on it. Seeing the "deluded" person whose "voices" command him to kill as similar to an automaton or robot—that is, an object that performs human-like motions but is not human—is a modern idea. Accepting the assertion of a "schizophrenic" that he killed his wife because God's voice commanded him to do so is not evidence of the validity of the explanation. In my view, such a person kills his victim because *that is what he wants to do*. But he disavows his intention; instead of acknowledging his motive, he defines himself as a helpless slave obeying orders. As I have shown elsewhere, the so-called voices some mentally ill people "hear" are their own inner voices or self-conversations, whose authorship they disown.[5] This interpretation is supported by the fact that neuroimaging studies of hallucinating persons reveal activation of Broca's (speech) area, not activation of Wernicke's (auditory) area.[6]

The "mental patient" who attributes his misdeed to "voices"—that is, to an agent other than himself, whose authority is irresistible—is not the victim of an irresistible impulse; he is an agent, a victimizer rationalizing his action by attributing it to an irresistible authority. The analogy between a person who "hears voices" and an object—say, a computer programmed to play chess—responding to information is false. Mental patients responding to the commands of "voices" resemble persons responding to the commands of authorities with irresistible powers, exemplified by suicide bombers who martyr themselves in the name of God. Both types of persons are moral agents, albeit both types represent themselves as slave-like objects, executing the wills of others (often identified as God or the devil). These representations are dramatic metaphors that actors and audience alike may, or may not, interpret as literal truths. It is not by accident that, in all of psychiatric literature, there is not a single account of voices that command a schizophrenic to be especially kind to his wife. That is because being kind to one's wife is not the sort of behavior to which we want to assign a causal (psychiatric) explanation.

The facile, but fallacious, equation of mental illness with mental incompetence precludes an empirically valid and logically consistent psychiatric explanation of behavior. For example, a patient's belief that his wife is a witch may be a metaphor (for thinking that she is a bad person) or a "delusion" (similar to a false/self-serving/destructive religious belief, such as Abraham's belief that it is God's wish that he sacrifice Isaac). We do not view the person who acts on the basis of false information (say, a wrong timetable) as having no reason for his action. Similarly, we ought not to view the person who acts on the basis of false belief ("delusion") as having no reason for his action. We may, as I noted, want to treat such a person as not blameworthy. However, that is not the same as asserting that he acts without reason or that his deed is "meaningless" or "senseless," the terms typically used to dismiss the meaning or sense of heinous crimes.

The typical mental patient is a conscious adult who has not been declared legally incompetent. "Seriously mentally disordered patients neither lack insight, nor is their competency impaired to the degree previously believed," writes George Hoyer, a professor at the Institute of Community Medicine, University of Tromse, Norway.[7] Moreover, mental patients are regularly considered competent to do some things but not others, for example, competent to live independently but not competent to reject psychiatric drug treatment; competent to stand trial but not competent to represent themselves in court; competent to vote but not competent to leave the hospital.[8]

Young children and senile persons engage, or may want to engage, in actions for which their reasons may be poor, indeed. But, again, that does not mean that their actions are not motivated by reasons. Bringing up children, "civilizing primitive people," forcibly converting people to the "true faith," rehabilitating criminals, and many other relations of domination-submission rest on the premise that the subject people's reasons for action are immature or erroneous and need to be "corrected" to enable them to enjoy "true freedom." As long as relations between psychiatrists and mental patients (especially "psychotics") rest on domination-submission, the idea of mental illness serves a similar set of functions: it explains the inferior person's (mis)behavior, exempts him from blame, and justifies his forcible control by psychiatrists.

"In 'The myth of mental illness,'" observed University of Sussex professor Rupert Wilkinson, "the psychiatrist Thomas Szasz . . . did identify an important process: we might call it 'a chase through language.' . . . Our better natures, it seems, introduce words to promote compassion—but residual needs to despise and distance weakness will not be stopped. . . . the terminology of mental illness substitutes labels of incompetence for labels of moral deficiency, and in a secular society this is no gift."[9]

IV

The word "mind" and the derivative term "mental illness" name two of our most important, but most confused and confusing, ideas. The Latin word *mens* means not only "mind" but also "intention" and "will," a signification still present in our use of the word "mind" as a verb. Because we attribute intention only to intelligent, sentient beings, minding implies agency.

The concept of mind—as the attribution of moral agency to some persons but not others—plays a crucial role in moral philosophy, law, and psychiatry. Infants and demented old persons cannot communicate by language and are therefore typically excluded from the category of moral agents. In the past, persons able to communicate by language—for example, slaves and women—were also denied the status of moral agents. Today, many children and mental patients—possessing the ability to communicate—are denied that status. The point is that attributing or refusing to attribute moral agency to the Other is a matter of both fact and tactic—a decision that depends not only on the Other's abilities but also on our attitude toward the Other. To be recognized as a moral agent, individuals must be able and willing to function as responsible members of society, and society must be willing to ascribe that capacity and status to them.

The dependence of moral agency on mindedness renders the judgment of impaired mindedness—that is, the diagnosis of "mental illness"—of paramount legal and social significance. Two common tactics characteristic of our age deserve special mention in this connection. One is treating persons as incompetent when in fact they are not—harming them under the guise of helping them. The other is treating persons as victims when in fact they are victimizers (of themselves or others)—excusing them of responsibility for their behavior (blaming their self-injury or injury of others on innocent third parties).

Paradoxically, the old, prescientific-religious explanation of human behavior is more faithful to the facts than the modern, scientific-psychiatric explanation of it. When we invent the Perfect Judge and call it "God," we create an arbiter who does not distinguish between two kinds of conduct—one rational, for which people are responsible, and another irrational, for which they are not. Being held responsible for our actions is what renders us fully human: it is the glory with which God endows everyone and the burden He imposes on everyone. Erroneous explanations of the material world lead to physical catastrophes, false explanations of the human condition, to moral catastrophes.

3

Might Makes the Metaphor

The South is dry and will vote dry. That is, everybody sober enough to
stagger to the polls will.

—Will Rogers (1879–1935)

RECENTLY (1973), I participated in one of those now-fashionable sym-
posia in which a group of well-known—at least among their colleagues—
psychiatrists reenact the drama of Babel: each in his own jargon—largely
incomprehensible to others—sets forth, in utter seriousness, the character,
cause, and cure of mental illness. The meeting was heavy on biology, with
elegant graphs and tables projected onto expensive screens demonstrating,
with irrefutable scientific evidence, the genetic basis of alcoholism and antisocial personality.

My presence at the occasion was, I suppose, a symptom of the "schizophrenia" now affecting the psychiatric establishment itself. I refer to the fact
that mental health professionals now display an equally intense interest in
the view that mental illnesses are baffling brain diseases and in the view that
their diagnostic labels are malicious medical metaphors.

I do not smoke and usually do not mind if others do. However, as I was
coming down with the flu at the time of this meeting, my throat was dry, and
I was undoubtedly more sensitive than I might otherwise have been to what I
was being exposed to—both through my ears and my nostrils. The intellectual
fare was not my dish. However, I felt that my colleagues were entitled to their
opinions. What I felt they were not entitled to was to proclaim that alcoholism
is a genetically determined mental disease and at the same time produce vast
quantities of smoke by steadily puffing on cigars, cigarettes, and pipes.

When my turn came to speak, I asked why, if alcoholism is a mental disease, is nicotinism not also a mental disease, and whether filling a room with

19

tobacco smoke might not be viewed as an antisocial act by those who don't smoke. The response was a ripple of applause from a small contingent of nonsmokers in the audience and a rising wave of anger and clouds of smoke directed toward me by my colleagues. Since the audience was composed mainly of psychiatrists and other mental health professionals, and since the members of these disciplines are especially fond of smoking, we nonsmokers were greatly outnumbered. As to my fellow panelists, they evidently felt that my remark did not deserve to be taken seriously: they did not answer my question and continued to smoke.

"Might," Plato asserted, "is right," thus offering one of the earliest and most often endorsed justifications of political justice. Since medicine, and especially psychiatry, is now even more politicized than law, it is time that we realize that might is also the power to make medical metaphors—called "psychiatric diagnoses." Psychiatrists speak of "alcoholism," regard it as a mental illness, and offer cures for it, but they do not speak of "nicotinism" and do not regard it as a disease. Indeed, there is now, in a Washington suburb, a much ballyhooed National Institute of Alcohol Abuse and Alcoholism, but there is no National Institute of Nicotine Abuse and Nicotinism. Isn't this because psychiatrists disapprove of alcoholism, but approve of and indeed encourage nicotinism by the most potent means of moral teaching in the world, namely, example? I submit that this inconsistency provides more insight into and understanding of what psychiatrists really mean by mental illness than the fakery and foolishness they now foist on the public under the guise of discoveries into the genetic causes and chemical cures of this "illness."

4

Diagnosis

From Description to Prescription

[T]o require medicine, said I, not merely for wounds or the incidence
of some seasonal maladies, but because of sloth . . . and compel the in-
genious sons of Asclepius to invent for diseases such names as fluxes and
flatulences, don't you think that disgraceful?

—Plato (428–348 BC), *The Republic*

I

NOSOLOGY, the scientific classification of diseases, is less than 200 years
old. It began with physicians dissecting corpses, comparing the abnormal
organs of persons who died of diseases with the normal organs of persons
who died in accidents or as a result of violence. And it was put on a scientific,
physical-chemical foundation by the German pathologist Rudolf Virchow
(1821–1902), whose definition of disease as a disturbance in the structure or
function of cells, tissues, and organs became the basis of classical nosology.

Until recently, the pathologist's diagnosis, which always trumped the
clinician's, was considered to be the correct name of the disease that ailed
or killed the patient. However, postwar developments in medical technology
and the provision of health care services shifted the focus of nosology from
postmortem to antemortem diagnoses, and from the patient's body to the
body politic.

The scientific diagnosis of live patients is, for the most part, a recent
technological development. The first diagnostic method, percussion, was
discovered in 1761 by Leopold Auenbrugger, the son of an innkeeper in
Graz, Austria. As a youngster he learned to tap caskets of wine to determine

21

the quantity of liquid in the container and applied the technique to the human chest. The systematic measurement of body temperature dates from 1852. The sphygmomanometer was invented in 1896. The more sophisticated tests used today are all twentieth-century developments.

Today, the identification of bodily abnormalities in living persons, making use of an array of sophisticated tools, is a highly developed science. The making of a clinical diagnosis—that is, identifying the lesion/disease (if there is one) to account for a living person's/patient's complaints/symptoms—is a technical routine requiring a standardized interpretation. Fifty years ago, some physicians were sought after because they were known as great diagnosticians. Today, there are no great diagnosticians. The sought-after physicians are now the great therapists, typically virtuoso surgeons or wizards of psychopharmacology.

Classic Virchowian nosology was the province of the pathologist, the expert on the postmortem examination of cadavers. In contrast, contemporary clinical nosology is the province partly of the medical administrator, the expert on Diagnosis Related Groups (DRGs), and partly of the medical-political activist, the expert on the costs and consequences of behaviors deemed to be diseases and of procedures deemed to be therapies.

II

The shift in nosological focus—from the human body to the body economic and body politic—is but one symptom of the pervasive politicization of medicine, redefined as the "delivery of health care." Reviewing the changing criteria for diagnosis, Yale pathologist Alvan R. Feinstein emphasizes the divergences among three systems—the International Classification of Diseases (ICD), the Problem-Oriented Record (POR), and the Diagnosis Related Group (DRG)—and states, "After magnificent scientific advances in etiological explanation and therapeutic intervention during the twentieth century, clinical medicine seems ready to enter the twenty-first century with a fundamental scientific defect in one of its oldest, most basic activities: the system used to identify and classify diseases."[1]

The problem to which Feinstein points is not a scientific imperfection but a moral defect. Current disease taxonomies are not intended to be, and often do not even pretend to be, scientific, that is, *descriptive*. Instead, they are political, that is, *prescriptive*. Their goal is not to identify bodily conditions that ought to be considered diseases but to create social policies, such as permitting and recommending the use of certain chemicals as safe and effective therapeutic agents, and prohibiting and punishing the use of others as medically worthless "drugs of abuse." A physician cogently observes, "The greatest danger with DRGs may result from linking monetary gain to the classification system, an idea supported by the current literature."[2] In my view, the new nosologies pose a much graver threat: by validating the politicization of medicine, they remove the last barriers against the medicalization of unwanted behaviors and thus pave the way for the unopposed, and unopposable, rule of the therapeutic state. Consider the following examples.

In November 1993, a group of investigators, supported in part by the Eli Lilly pharmaceutical company, estimated "that the annual costs of depression in the United States total approximately $43.7 billion."[3] Mental health advocates frequently cite this figure and others like it, *as if it proved that depression is a disease*. For instance, Tipper Gore, mental health advisor to President Clinton's Health Care Task Force, asserts that "depression alone costs society $43.7 billion annually . . . Lithium has saved the economy billions of dollars over the past two decades, and Clozapine now allows many of the most seriously ill to live their lives productively."[4] Psychiatrist Jose M. Santiago explains: "[D]epression is an illness that merits urgent attention by health-care policy reformers as its costs to society are considerable."[5]

The view that certain chemicals enhance productivity is hardly a new idea. South American Indians have long chewed coca leaves for this reason. Freud felt that smoking enabled him to be more creative. He did not claim, however, that the beneficial effect of nicotine is evidence that the smoker suffers from a disease for which nicotine is a treatment. Basing the claim for the disease status for depression and schizophrenia on the subject's allegedly favorable response to drugs rests on precisely that logic. If giving a particular drug is authoritatively classified as a "treatment," the subject as a "patient," and his posttreatment behavior as an "improvement," then, ipso facto, the dis-ease that he had was a bona fide disease. Thus has "response to treatment" become one of our diagnostic criteria.

The logic is circular: The popularity of Prozac is evidence that depression is common, and FDA approval of this drug and of other so-called antidepressants proves that depression is a disease. In the absence of objective criteria for diagnosing depression, there is heated debate about who should take antidepressant drugs. Here is the politically correct answer to this question: "[U]nlike, say, high cholesterol levels, which show up in laboratory tests, the diagnosis of depression is often subjective. What do you use as criteria? . . . Maybe an individual is not clinically depressed, but he or she still feels depressed and goes to the physician 15 times a year and misses 30 days of work. . . . If the individual takes the drug and doesn't go to the physician and doesn't miss any work, the benefit to the total health care cost would be there."[6]

In a similar vein, the *New York Times* informs us, "At least 11 million Americans have a bout of depression every year, and only about 30 percent currently get medication that could help them. . . . Many millions more whose symptoms don't amount to clinical depression might also look to such drugs." The adjective "clinical" is a code word justifying drug treatment and, if need be, involuntary psychiatric interventions. The fact that not a single textbook of pathology recognizes depression and schizophrenia as diseases has not in the least dampened popular and political enthusiasm for their diagnosis and treatment.[7]

Tipper Gore insists that "antidepressants such as Prozac have been developed for the treatment of diagnosable mental illnesses, not the casual pursuit of 'happiness.'"[8] The term "diagnosable" is here a code word that means "government-approved and insurance-reimbursable." Gore's protest is superfluous. As everyone knows, the pursuit of happiness by means of government-disapproved drugs is now punished more severely than violent crime. The minimum penalty imposed by U.S. federal law for "attempted murder with harm" is 6.5 years; for possession of LSD, it is 10.1 years.[9] In addition, possessing an illegal drug is presumptive evidence of using it, being addicted to it, and hence having a disease as well.

III

Defining the use of drugs disapproved by the state as a disease (substance abuse, chemical dependency, addiction), and the use of drugs approved by the state as a treatment (antabuse, methadone, Haldol), illustrates the radical politicization of both nosology and therapy. If the government validates a drug, bestowing on it FDA approval for the treatment of, say, X, then, ipso facto, X is accepted as a disease, for example, attention hyperactivity disorder, clinical depression, panic attack. In other words, if there is a drug to treat "it," then "it" must be a disease. Illustrative is the report of the Johnson and Johnson pharmaceutical company having "won federal approval for its schizophrenia drug Risperdal, which has caused a stir among doctors and patients seeking new treatments for one of the most devastating and expensive of all illnesses. . . . The disease costs $33 billion annually in the U.S."[10]

Brandishing such enormous costs makes it a taboo to question whether schizophrenia is a disease and whether antipsychotic drugs help patients. At the same time, the dogmatic view that mental diseases are brain diseases, treatable with chemicals, dehumanizes the denominated patients. Individuals diagnosed schizophrenic and their behavior disappear into a fog of literalized metaphors. One psychiatrist who studied Risperdal explained "how research found it treated schizophrenia's delusions better than haloperidol, one of the most widely used antipsychotic drugs."[11] Who cares that schizophrenia cannot have delusions? That having delusions is not like having diabetes, because what the observer calls "delusion," the subject calls "belief"? That antischizophrenia drugs, eagerly embraced by the patients' familial and psychiatric adversaries, are regularly rejected by the patients whose suffering they allegedly relieve? Declared Laurie Flynn of the National Alliance for the Mentally Ill, "This new drug means a whole new group of people will have an opportunity to return to productive life."[12] Who cares whether this a serious forecast or a self-serving exaggeration?

IV

Before World War II, few diseases were treatable, but nosology was an honest enterprise. Now, many diseases are treatable, but nosology is a dishonest enterprise. The old nosology, whose aims were empirical validity and scientific respectability, was unconcerned with the treatment of diseases. The new nosology, whose aims are political favor and professional profit, rests on arrogant claims about treatability as a criterion of illness.

Virchowian nosology was an offspring of nineteenth-century science and the free market. Except for psychiatry and public health, medicine was then economically and politically independent of the state. Today, the definitions of disease and treatment are controlled by a monopolistic alliance of medicine and the state; health care is viewed as an entitlement; and physicians, endorsing neuromythological fantasies about mental illnesses, join the mindless political chatter about nonexistent market forces in medicine.

In short, we are in the process of replacing the classic empirical-pathological criteria of disease with new political-economic criteria of it. Current nosology no longer encodes the objectively verifiable condition of patients' bodies. Instead, it reflects the attitudes of their family and society to their idleness, lack of productivity, and dependence and their families' justifications for the interventions they want politicians to legitimize, and psychiatrists to impose on them, as therapy.

5

Diagnoses Are Not Diseases

Learn to recognize the symptoms of MENTAL ILLNESS. Schizophre-
nia, Manic Depression and Severe Depression are BRAIN DISEASES.
—Hawaii State Alliance for the
Mentally Ill (1991)

I

IN 1980, the American Psychiatric Association (APA) published the third
edition of its *Diagnostic and Statistical Manual of Mental Disorders* (*DSM-
III*).[1] This document was celebrated for its deletion of homosexuality from
the list of mental disorders and was hailed as the symbol of the new, "medical" psychiatry. Yet only three years later, ostensibly because "data were
emerging from new studies that were inconsistent with some of the diagnostic criteria," the APA embarked on a revision of *DSM-III*.[2] In 1987, *DSM-
III-R* was published. A year later, the board of trustees of the APA appointed
a task force to prepare *DSM-IV*. In 1991, the APA published *DSM-IV Options Books: Work in Progress*.[3] More than ever, the profession of psychiatry
is determined to ground its medical legitimacy on creating diagnoses and
pretending that they are diseases.

II

Intrigued by the patently metaphoric character of the psychiatric vocabulary, which, nevertheless, is widely recognized and validated as a legitimate
medical idiom, I decided, at the very beginning of my professional career,
to explore the nature and function of these literalized metaphors and to
expose them, as metaphors, to the light of public scrutiny.[4] I thus managed

to set in motion a controversy about mental illness that is still raging, and whose crux is still often misunderstood. Scientists, jurists, mental health professionals, and laypeople alike seem to believe that the demonstration of a genetic defect said to be causing a mental illness (for example, alcoholism), or a lesion in the brains of mental patients (for example, schizophrenics), would prove, or has already proved, that mental illnesses exist and are "like other illnesses." This is not so. If mental illnesses are diseases of the central nervous system (for example, paresis), then they are diseases of the brain, not the mind; and if mental illnesses are the names of (mis)behaviors (for example, fear and avoidance of narrow spaces, called "claustrophobia"), then they are behaviors, not diseases. A screwdriver may be a drink or an implement. No amount of research on orange juice and vodka can establish that it is a hitherto unrecognized form of a carpenter's tool.

Although such linguistic clarification is useful for individuals who want to think clearly, it is not useful for people whose social institutions rest on the unexamined, literal use of their master metaphors. Accordingly, I have long maintained that psychiatric metaphors play the same role in our therapeutic society that religious metaphors have played and continue to play in theological societies. For example, both Christianity and Islam affirm the existence of a life after death, and many people say they believe in such a life. The fact that many more Americans believe in the existence of heaven than in the existence of hell tells us more, of course, about Americans than about life after death. However, if we use the term *life* to denote the biological lives of human beings, then, literally speaking, life is a process that has a beginning, called "conception" or "birth," and an end, called "death." The phrase "life after death" is, therefore, an oxymoron. Still, if a person believes in life after death, his conviction is not likely to be dispelled by pointing this out to him. Because the idea of life after death makes many people feel better, and because "You cannot prove there is 'nothing' after death," as true believers put it, those who believe in life after death and those who do not have nothing more to say to each other on this subject. The same goes for the colloquy between those who believe in mental illness and those who do not.

While there is a large common ground between the images of heaven-hell and sanity-insanity, there is also a difference between them that must be noted. For any living person, his own death is, by definition, a future event.

In this sense, it is true that none of us can know what will happen to him after he dies. On the other hand, the terms "mental health" and "mental illness" refer to behaviors displayed by living human beings. And we know perfectly well what these terms signify: approved and disapproved, legitimate and illegitimate ways of living *life before death*. Thus, everyone one of us makes certain basic choices. For example, either we accept that life is finite and ends in death, or we reject this view and embrace the belief in a life after death. Similarly, either we accept life as an unceasing struggle for meaning, legitimacy, and other values that inexorably bring people into conflict with others and themselves, and in which individuals can succeed and fail, or we reject this view and believe that there is a mentally healthy state the attainment of which would eliminate human strife and personal failure.

Religion is, among other things, the institutionalized denial of the finiteness of life; individuals who want to reject the reality of death can thus theologize life and entrust its management to clerical professionals. Similarly, psychiatry is, among other things, the institutionalized denial of the tragic nature of life; individuals who want to reject the reality of free will and responsibility can thus medicalize life and entrust its management to health professionals. Marx was close to the mark when he asserted that "Religion is the opiate of the people." But religion is not the opiate of the people; the human mind is. After all, religion is a product of our own minds, and so, too, is psychiatry. In short, the mind is its own opiate. And its ultimate drug is the Word.

Despite such considerations, an editorial in the prestigious British medical journal *Lancet* remains fixated on the mirage of finding the cause of schizophrenia, like that of paresis, in the brain. Lamenting the state of psychiatry 150 years after the founding of the (British) Association of Medical Officers of Asylums and Hospitals for the Insane—which, after some intermediary name changes became, in 1971, the Royal College of Psychiatrists—the editorial writer states, "What about psychiatric research? We seem to be no closer to finding the real, presumed biological, causes of the major psychiatric illnesses. . . . This is not to decry the value of such research—if the causes of conditions such as . . . schizophrenia are found it will be an advance of the same magnitude as the identification of the syphilis spirochaete in the brains of patients with general paralysis of the insane."[5]

As I mentioned, I took up the profession of psychiatry in part to debunk the biological-reductionist impulse that motivated its origin and that continues to fuel its engines; in other words, to combat the contention, and to refute the expectation, that abnormal behaviors must be understood as the products of abnormal brains. Ironically, it was easier to do this then, more than sixty years ago, than today. For the better part of three centuries, the idea that every phenomenon named a "mental illness" will prove to be a bona fide brain disease was a hypothesis that could be supported or opposed. However, after the 1960s, this hypothesis became increasingly accepted as a scientific fact, like the spherical shape of the earth. Of course, it is still physically possible and legally permissible to say that mental illnesses do not exist. But since only a charlatan, a fool, or a fanatic disputes facts or opposes science, such a critic is likely to be dismissed as irrational or worse.

Thus, for the moment at least, psychiatrists and their powerful allies have seemingly succeeded in persuading the scientific community, the courts, the media, and the general public that the conditions they call "mental disorders" are diseases—that is to say, phenomena independent of human motivation or will. This is a curious development, for, until recently, only psychiatrists—who know little about medicine and less about science—embraced such blind physical reductionism. Most scientists knew better. Michael Polanyi's remarks, in an essay aptly titled "Life's Irreducible Structures," are illustrative. In 1968, he wrote, "We can see then that, though rooted in the body, the mind is free in its actions—exactly as our common sense knows it to be free. The mind harnesses neurophysiological mechanisms; though it depends on them, it is not determined by them."[6]

Anticipating already then that such a view would expose him to accusations of being antiscientific, Polanyi went on to reemphasize that the mark of the true scientist is not making grandiose theoretical claims or flamboyant promises of impending therapeutic triumphs, but accepting limits and building on the possible: "The recognition of certain basic impossibilities has laid the foundations of some major principles of physics and chemistry; similarly, recognition of the impossibility of understanding living things in terms of physics and chemistry, far from setting limits to our understanding of life, will guide it in the right direction."[7]

IV

It is not by accident that the more firmly psychiatrically inspired ideas take hold of the collective American mind, the more foolishness and injustice they generate. The specifications of the Americans with Disabilities Act (ADA), a federal law enacted in 1990, is a case in point.

The official aim of the law is "to diminish the stigma of mental illness and reduce discrimination involving . . . at least 60 million Americans, between the ages of 18 and 64, [who] will experience a mental disorder during their lifetimes."[8] If this is the politically and psychiatrically correct view, how can I maintain that there are no mental disorders? Not very easily. But, then, Will Rogers can be summoned for help. "Compared to those fellows in Congress," he wrote, "I'm just an amateur. . . . [E]very time they make a joke, it's a law! and every time they make a law, it's a joke."[9] The Americans with Disabilities Act is a law, but that does not prevent it from being a joke—and a very bad one, at that.

Long ago, our lawmakers acquiesced in letting psychiatrists literalize the metaphor of mental illness. Having accepted fictitious mental diseases as facts, they now had to identify which of these manufactured maladies were covered, and which were not covered, under the ADA. They had no trouble doing so, creating a veritable DSM-Congress—that is, a list of congressionally accredited mental diseases. Thus, the ADA covers "claustrophobia, personality problems, and mental retardation; [but does not cover] kleptomania, pyromania, compulsive gambling, and . . . transvestism."[10] Well, at least Congress agrees with me that stealing, setting fires, gambling, and cross-dressing are not diseases. But it is positively comical that our senators and congressmen do not realize that they have no more ground for excluding these alleged disorders from ADA coverage than they have for including those that they accept for coverage.

At about the same time as the *New York Times* and the *Wall Street Journal* published major reports on the "New Deal for the Mentally Ill,"[11] the *American Journal of Psychiatry* (the American Psychiatric Association's official journal) published a feature article on kleptomania.[12] In keeping with the *DSM-III-R*, the author's *premise* was that kleptomania is a bona fide illness. His task was simply to explore and document its incidence, character, and cause. Not surprisingly, the author's principal conclusion was to propose "a biopsychosocial model of the *etiology* of kleptomania . . . [that] emphasizes possible childhood abuse as a precipitating factor. . . . "[13] Perhaps I should add here that the American Psychiatric Association recognizes claustrophobia (which the ADA accepts as a mental illness) and kleptomania (which the ADA rejects) as mental disorders on exactly the same footing.

V

It is not my intention to discuss here what we mean when we use the word "disease." However, apropos of the ADA and its exclusion of kleptomania, I want to note that, as normal users of English, we do not attribute motives to diseases, and do not call motivated actions (bodily) "diseases." For example, we attribute no motive to a person for having leukemia; it would be foolish to say that a particular motive led to a person's having glaucoma; and it would be quite nonsensical to assert that an illness (say, diabetes) caused a person to become a senator. In short, one of the most important philosophical-political features of the concept of mental illness is that, at one fell swoop, it removes motivation from action, adds it to illness, and thus destroys the very possibility of separating disease from nondisease.[14] This crucial function of the idea of mental illness is dramatically illustrated by the psychiatrists' definition of certain acts of stealing as a disease (kleptomania); by the media's acceptance of this behavior as a disease, even when the act is called "shoplifting"; and by the mental health professionals' explanations of the "causes" that allegedly result in this disease.

In a newspaper report on shoplifting as a disease, the director of Onondaga (New York) County's Drinking and Driving Program explains: "Syracuse needs Shoplifters Anonymous. . . . There are more than 3,000 arrests for shoplifting in Onondaga County. It's costing everyone a fortune."[15] Although the program is described as "voluntary," it is in fact a substitute for a criminal penalty: "If the thief completes the course, the arrest vanishes from his or her record." The report illustrates that experts and media alike treat shoplifting as a disease, to which they nevertheless then attribute various motives. In the treatment program, the shoplifters "learn *why* they steal . . . there are several *reasons why* people shoplift: They feel entitled. Perhaps they feel prices are too high; they are angry at authority. . . . It's a mental health problem."[16]

Another article, a few days later, was devoted to explaining "shopping addiction," which was defined "as a situation where a person may utilize shopping as an activity to change their [*sic*] mood."[17] Such a person "really doesn't like shopping. It's not a free experience, because it has a very driven quality to it." The experts cited do not even pretend to present pathological (anatomic or physiological) evidence to support their claim; instead, they drop the names of "famous addicted shoppers . . . [such as] Princess Diana, Jacqueline Kennedy Onassis, and Imelda Marcos," ostensibly as proof that shopaholism is a disease. Is addiction to shopping "treatable," the reporter inquires. "Yes, but with variable results, say the experts. . . . The treatment is very much like any other addiction . . . you have to look at it as a life-long process."[18] Cui bono?

VI

Although Congress has so far remained unconvinced that the behavior we call "shoplifting"—but psychiatrists call "kleptomania"—is an illness, it might be of interest to list here just a few of the behaviors for which psychiatrists have disease names and that the ADA implicitly accepts as bona fide diseases, on equal footing with, say, malaria and melanoma:

> 300.70 BODY DYSMORPHIC DISORDER (DYSMORPHOPHOBIA). The essential feature of this disorder is preoccupation with some imagined defect in appearance in a normal-appearing person.[19]
>
> 300.14 MULTIPLE PERSONALITY DISORDER. The essential feature of this disorder is the existence within the person of two or more distinct personalities . . . At least two of the personalities, at some time and recurrently, take full control of the person's behavior.[20]
>
> 302.89 FROTTEURISM. The essential feature of this disorder is recurrent, intense, sexual urges and sexually arousing fantasies, of at least six months' duration, involving touching and rubbing against a nonconsenting person.[21]

> 302.71 HYPOACTIVE SEXUAL DESIRE DISORDER. Persistently or recurrently deficient or absent sexual fantasies and desire for sexual activity. The judgment of deficiency or absence is made by the clinician.[22]
>
> 301.51 FACTITIOUS DISORDER WITH PHYSICAL SYMPTOMS. The essential feature of this disorder is the intentional production of physical symptoms. The presentation may be a total fabrication, as in complaints of acute abdominal pain in the absence of any such pain.[23]

VII

The political and popular acceptance of such and similar psychiatric words and phrases as medical terms generates a steady stream of absurd situations. Nevertheless, because we regard psychiatric dispositions as humane and useful, neither the erroneous nature of psychiatric premises nor the injustice of psychiatric dispositions discredits psychiatry as a medical specialty. Consider the following story, typical of what now passes as psychiatric explanation and legal judgment.

A forty-two-year-old female orthopedic surgeon, working in a Virginia suburb of Washington, D.C., is arrested for drunken driving. She resists arrest, refuses to take a breath or blood test, curses and kicks the police. Taken into custody, she finally consents to take a breath test and registers 0.13, over the 0.10 legal limit for blood alcohol. "At trial she maintained that the circumstances of her behavior at the time of her arrest were a result of PMS [premenstrual syndrome]." She was acquitted.[24]

In reporting this story in *Psychiatric News,* the American Psychiatric Association's biweekly newspaper, the writer asks, "Does LLPDD [late luteal phase dysphoric disorder] exist?" The same question might be raised, of course, about every non-bodily disease. The reporter then cites the comments of several psychiatrists that illustrate dramatically psychiatry's intellectual bankruptcy and moral desolation: "The decision as to whether or not LLPDD will be assigned its own diagnostic category in the fourth edition of APA's *Diagnostic and Statistical Manual of Mental Disorders* (DSM-IV) is 'a political land mine,' according to Allen Frances, M.D., chair of the Task Force on DSM-IV."[25] David Rubinow, MD, a psychiatrist who "has done research at NIH on PMS for more than a decade," offered this opinion: "As far as I am concerned, the decision to include PMS in DSM-IV will be made on political rather than medical considerations. . . . It's quite clear there are a substantial number of people with PMS who never get arrested. To attribute guilt in a crime to PMS is a somewhat hazardous enterprise."[26]

Precisely the same argument can be made about any mental illness used to support an insanity defense. John W. Hinckley Jr. was acquitted of shooting President Reagan because psychiatrists testified he had schizophrenia. But how many people diagnosed as schizophrenic shoot a president? And of those who do, how many claim they did it to impress Jody Foster? Actually, Hinckley's act was a unique performance that, in some ways, may be more revealing of the actor's character than his ordinary behaviors, performed routinely. Psychiatrists deny this, as indeed they must, because they realize that their entire enterprise hinges on society's acceptance of the proposition that human beings diagnosed as mentally ill have a brain disease that deprives them of free will.

VIII

I have offered these reflections in a further effort to clarify the crucial differences between diseases and diagnoses. Diseases, in the old-fashioned, literal sense of the term, occur naturally—like avalanches or earthquakes; whereas diagnoses are man-made artifacts or constructs—like books or bridges. Which raises the question: Why do we make diagnoses? We have several reasons for doing so:

1. Scientific: to identify the organs or tissues affected and perhaps the cause of the illness.

2. Professional: to enlarge the scope, and thus the power and prestige of a state-protected medical monopoly and the income of its practitioners.

3. Legal: to justify state-sanctioned coercive interventions outside of the criminal justice system.

4. Political-economic: to justify enacting and enforcing measures aimed at promoting public health and providing funds for research and treatment on projects classified as medical.

5. Personal: To enlist the support of public opinion, the media, and the legal system for bestowing special privileges (and impose special hardships) on persons diagnosed as (mentally) ill.

It is not by coincidence that most psychiatric diagnoses are twentieth-century inventions. The aim of the classic, nineteenth-century model of diagnosis was to identify bodily lesions (diseases) and their material causes (etiology). For example, the term "pneumococcal pneumonia" identifies the organ affected, the lungs, and the cause of the illness, infection with the pneumococcus.[27] Pneumococcal pneumonia is an example of a pathology-driven diagnosis. Diagnoses driven by other motives—such as the desire to coerce the patient or to secure government funding for the treatment of the illness—generate different diagnostic constructions and lead to different conceptions of disease. Today, of course, even diagnoses of what used to be strictly medical diseases are no longer principally pathology-driven. Because of third-party funding of hospital costs and physicians' fees, even the diagnoses of persons suffering from bona fide illnesses—for example, asthma or arthritis—are utterly distorted by economic considerations. In fact, final diagnoses on the discharge summaries of hospitalized patients are often no longer made by physicians, but by bureaucrats skilled in the ways of Medicare, Medicaid, and private health insurance reimbursement (based partly on what ails the patient, and partly on which medical terms for his ailment and treatment ensure the most generous reimbursement for the services rendered to him). As for psychiatry, it ought to be clear that, except for the diagnoses of neurological diseases (which are treated by neurologists), no psychiatric diagnosis is, or can be, pathology-driven; instead, all such diagnoses are driven by nonmedical—that is, economic, personal, legal, political, and social—considerations or incentives. Accordingly, psychiatric diagnoses point neither to patho-anatomic or patho-physiological lesions, nor to disease-causative agents, but to human behaviors and human problems, and to the fallible attempts of fallible moral agents to cope with problematic human behaviors.

6

The Existential Identity Thief

Falsehood flies and the truth comes limping after; so that when men come
to be undeceived it is too late: the jest is over and the tale has had its effect.
—Jonathan Swift (1667–1745),
The Examiner (1710)

I

ONE OF THE BASIC FUNCTIONS of living organisms is avoiding danger.
In human beings, the emotion of fear serves that function. Because feeling
fear is unpleasant, we try to escape it by seeking protection from danger, typically by looking to a protector to protect us. Tragically, this longing—be it for
a deity, demagogue, dictator, or doctor—is, itself, a source of danger. "Necessity," William Pitt (1759–1806) famously remarked, "is the plea for every infringement of human freedom. It is the argument of tyrants; it is the creed of
slaves." (Pitt was prime minister of Britain twice, 1783–1801 and 1804–6.)

Fear of the insane and the psychiatrist's role as society's protector from
the risk someone so described allegedly poses is what has made the mere as-
cription of the label "insane" a justification for depriving the bearer of liberty.
Although the idea of "the dangerous madman" is a bugaboo or a tautology
(because we redefine bad as mad, deviant as deranged), it has captivated the
contemporary mind—secular and religious alike—and has entrapped some of
the most admired modern intellectuals.

II

In *A History of Western Philosophy*, Bertrand Russell (1872–1970), the great
atheist skeptic, tried to refute David Hume's skeptical empiricism and concluded that he was unequal to the task:

It is therefore important to discover whether there is any answer to Hume within the framework of a philosophy that is wholly or mainly empirical. If not, there is no intellectual difference between sanity and insanity. The lunatic who believes that he is a poached egg is to be condemned solely on the ground that he is in a minority, or rather—since we must not assume democracy—on the ground that the government does not agree with him. This is a desperate point of view, and it must be hoped that there is some way of escaping from it.[1]

Russell's "desperation" was inconsistent with his skepticism, expressed earlier in his *Sceptical Essays,* where he had stated, "I wish to propose for the reader's favourable consideration a doctrine . . . that it is undesirable to believe a proposition when there is no ground whatever for supposing it true."[2] Russell was skeptical about religion but not about psychiatry. Positing the existence of a "lunatic who believes that he is a poached egg" is a perfect example of believing "a proposition when there is no ground whatever for supposing it to be true."

Clive Staples Lewis (1898–1963), the celebrated Christian apologist, believed in religion but disbelieved in psychiatry. Nevertheless, in his famous "trilemma," he too used the imaginary poached-egg man to support his reason for believing in the divinity of Jesus:

I am trying here to prevent anyone saying the really foolish thing that people often say about Him: "I'm ready to accept Jesus as a great moral teacher, but I don't accept His claim to be God." That is the one thing we must not say. A man who was merely a man and said the sort of things Jesus said would not be a great moral teacher. He would be either a lunatic—on a level with the man who says he is a poached egg—or else he would be the Devil of Hell. You must make your choice. Either this man was, and is, the Son of God: or else a madman or something worse. You can shut Him up for a fool, you can spit at Him and kill Him as a demon; or you can fall at His feet and call Him Lord and God. But let us not come with any patronising nonsense about His being a great human teacher. He has not left that open to us.[3]

The model lunatic as a person who believes himself to be a poached egg evidently was fashionable among twentieth-century English academics, at least at Oxbridge. Let us scrutinize this modern psychiatric miracle.

III

In a debate unrelated to matters psychiatric, Russell, the hard-headed empiricist, would emphasize that we have no way of knowing what a person believes himself to be. We can know only what he tells us about who or what he is and have no grounds for treating his claim as, a priori, true.

In ordinary English as well as in the idiom of psychiatry, we call a person's claim that he is a poached egg a "delusion." I have seen many persons with so-called delusions and have read about many more, but have never seen or read of a poached-egg man. In nineteenth-century European asylums, the most popular delusion was being Napoleon. In modern American mental hospitals, it is being Jesus. Whether or not the speaker believes his delusion to be true is irrelevant. The simplest, most parsimonious explanation for his speech act is that he is lying. In his *Sceptical Essays,* Russell himself suggested this interpretation. He wrote:

> A man who has suffered some humiliation invents a theory that he is King
> of England, and develops all kinds of ingenious explanations of the fact that
> he is not treated with that respect which his exalted position demands. In
> this case, his delusion is one with which his neighbors do not sympathize,
> so they lock him up. But if, instead of asserting only his own greatness, he
> asserts the greatness of his nation or his class or his creed, he wins hosts of
> adherents, and becomes a political or religious leader. (1)

IV

People often claim or pretend to be someone they are not. When they do it on the stage, we call their behavior "acting." When they impersonate another for economic gain, defrauding others in the process, we call it "identity theft." We treat them as criminals, guilty of committing fraud, not as lunatics harboring false beliefs. When, however, an individual impersonates, say, Jesus, we refuse to see the self-evident method in his madness, the desire to gain existential rather than economic advantage, and dismiss his conduct as "meaningless delusion." I submit that we ought to view such behavior as a type of "existential identity theft," a phenomenon that presents no particular challenge to either philosophy or theology. Yet Russell and Lewis both regarded the existential identity thief as presenting the grandest of philosophical and theological problems. Russell spoke of it as "a desperate point of view, and it must be hoped that there is some way of escaping from it." Lewis declared, "*Either this man was, and is, the Son of God: or else a madman or something worse.*" There is an obvious third choice.

The man who says he is a poached egg is a liar, and that ought to be the end of the matter, for theology, philosophy, and psychiatry alike. If we prefer to cast Lewis's riddle in softer terms, we might say that the man in Nazareth 2,000 years ago who said he is the son of God was a god-obsessed Jew, using a figurative language fashionable at the time, expressing and conveying a meaning to himself and others the exact signification of which we have no way of recapturing. Much as I admire Lewis the man and his many memorable books, his assertion about Jesus—"You can shut Him up for a fool, you can spit at Him and kill Him as a demon; or you can fall at His feet and call Him Lord and God. But let us not come with any patronising nonsense about His being a great human teacher. He has not left that open to us"—is simplistic and foolish. Lewis said that his aim was to show us why we ought to believe in the divinity of Jesus. Accepting his own postulate, he asserted that this hypothetical man-god had forbidden us to say "patronising nonsense" about him and that we must obey his prohibition. In short, Lewis treated his premise as proof of itself.

For the man who says he is Jesus, his identity thievery is an existential coup. For psychiatry, such a man—Jesus or poached egg—is an existential and economic gold mine. The fact that modern societies choose to value the products of this "salted mine" more highly than gold, indeed that they revere it as the science and practice of psychiatry, is another issue.

Finally, both Russell and Lewis compounded their mistaken reasoning about the nature of existential identity theft by assuming that individuals or society need to sanction the thief. Russell declared, "The lunatic who believes that he is a poached egg is to be condemned solely on the ground that he is in a minority, . . . etc." Lewis agreed: "You can shut Him [Jesus as liar] up for a fool . . . " These are non sequiturs. There is no need for individuals or society to condemn and punish the existential identity thief. Severing relations with him suffices for our self-protection.

7

Defining Disease

In our time it is the physician who exercises the cure of souls. . . . And he knows what to do.

[Doctor]: "You must travel to a watering-place, and then must keep riding a horse . . . and then diversion, diversion, plenty of diversion . . . "

[Patient]: "To relieve an anxious conscience?"

[Doctor]: "Bosh! Get out with that stuff! An anxious conscience! No such thing exists any more."

—Søren Kierkegaard (1813–1855), "A Visit to the Doctor: Can Medicine Abolish the Anxious Conscience?" in *Parables of Kierkegaard*

I

ILLNESS AND HEALING are as old as civilization. For millennia, the shaman or priest sought to help persons suffering from all manner of human adversities, only some of which do we now regard as diseases. Distinguishing between sin and sickness, between faith healing and medical treatment was a slow historical process, still incomplete in the minds and lives of millions. The scientific-materialist approach to medical healing—a western European idea—is less than two hundred years old.

Traditionally, the physician was a private entrepreneur. In the United States, only in the twentieth century did the federal and state governments begin to regulate and restrict the sale of drugs and the practice of medicine. After the end of World War II (earlier in the Soviet Union), the distribution of medical services throughout the developed world was transformed from a capitalist to a socialist system: the source of the physician's income shifted from the patient to the government or a government-regulated insurance system. At the same time, more and more personal habits and problems—from smoking to obesity to the management of unruly children—became defined as diseases, and more and more drugs were removed from the free market and made available only by prescription, only to persons diagnosed as ill and called "patients." Western societies were transformed from theocracies to democracies and then to pharmacracies.[1]

What should, and what should not, count as a disease? is a troubling question for all of medicine and especially for psychiatry. Everyone—doctors and patients, politicians and people—has a stake in how we demarcate disease from nondisease. None of us can escape the obligation to grapple with and decide how and where to draw this line. The question requires two different answers—one to satisfy the needs of medical science, another to satisfy the needs of medical practice and the persons it serves.

Medical science, a part of natural science, is concerned with the empirical investigation of the material world—the human body—by means of precisely defined and rigorously applied concepts and techniques. Medical practice, though based on science and the use of scientific technology, is not a science: it is a type of human service, the content and delivery of which are shaped by economic, ideological, religious, and political interests. In the delivery of medical care, insistence on similar precision and rigor is condemned as rigidity and lack of compassion.

The conflict between the need for precision and rigor in practicing science and the need for flexibility and compassion in providing medical care is reflected in our current nosology—a mixture of precisely identified natural phenomena and imprecisely defined economic, ideological, political, and social judgments and occurrences. As a result, this classification system is an intellectual embarrassment and an invitation to political-economic mischief. Extricating ourselves from the dilemmas of contemporary health care policy and politics requires that we acknowledge the need for two (or more) systems of defining and classifying diseases.

Science is synonymous with materialism, with the study of facts, with how things are. It is axiomatic that there can be no scientific investigation or scientific theory of nonmaterial "entities" and moral concepts such as angel and devil, spirit and mind, virtue and vice. To say that is not the same as saying that those things "do not exist." They "exist," but they are not a part of the material world. Their study entails inquiry into and reasoning about not facts but beliefs (explanations), experiences (how things feel), values (good and bad), and social policies (what actions in what circumstances ought to be considered licit and illicit).

All this is commonplace. Nevertheless, prominent medical scientists and prestigious publications regularly ignore, overlook, and obscure that we use, and need to use, the concept of disease both as a value-neutral scientific term to describe and explain aspects of the material world and as a value-laden ethical term to identify, excuse, condemn, and justify (nonmaterial) human aspirations, laws, and customs; and that we ought to distinguish clearly and honestly between these two different meanings and uses of the term.

II

For the greater part of two thousand years, from the days of Hippocrates (c. 460–380 BC) until the Enlightenment, physicians and philosophers believed that diseases were caused by disturbances of four basic elements, called "humors": blood, phlegm, yellow bile, and black bile. Each humor was associated with a major organ of the body, as anatomy—influenced by astrology rather than by dissection—was then understood. Blood related to the heart, phlegm to the brain, yellow bile to the liver, and black bile to the spleen. Treatment consisted of methods presumed to restore humoral balance. Outgrowing old ideas is a gradual process. It is possible, however, to fix two dates that decisively mark the beginning of a new age in the definition, identification, and understanding of bodily diseases and of physical elements of which they are composed. In 1858, the German pathologist Rudolf Virchow (1821–1902) published his thesis *Cellular Pathology as Based upon Physiological and Pathological Histology*. For the next century, the standard scientific measure—the "gold standard"—of disease was bodily lesion, objectively identifiable by anatomical, physiological, or other physico-chemical observation or measurement. In 1869, the Russian chemist Dimitri Mendeleyev (1834–1907) published his epoch-making paper, "The Relation between the Properties and Atomic Weights of the Elements." This was the first formulation of the periodic table of elements, a scheme that not only provided a precise identification of all known elements, but also identified elements not yet known whose existence Mendeleyev's theory postulated and predicted.

To disease as pathological lesion and to the periodic table as a list of physical elements, I suggest that we add here gold as a monetary standard. Why? Because these three systems exemplify ordering our world by precise and objective criteria *independent of human desire, moral judgment, or political power.* Institutions and individuals aspiring to exercise control over our personal lives—church and state, politicians and physicians—have always experienced, and continue to experience, independence from them as an impertinence, an interference with their "sacred duty" to govern and "serve the public interest." Not surprisingly, the security of fixed monetary and medical standards has been imperiled from the start. From ancient despots to the political leaders of modern democracies, rulers have sought monopolistic control over the monetary system. Modern therapeutic states assume similar monopolistic control over defining diseases and treatments.[2]

III

Modern societies are profoundly dependent on the hard sciences and the technologies they create and sustain. Therefore, modern states—with a few interesting but practically insignificant exceptions, such as Lysenkoism in the Soviet Union and Aryan physics in Nazi Germany—have abstained from using their power to destroy the objective criteria and empirical methods of science. With respect to money and medicine, in contrast, modern Western states have exercised no such restraint. Just the opposite: they have delegitimized and destroyed both the gold monetary standard and gold medical standard. Why? Because these systems exemplify ordering our world by precise and objective criteria *independent of human desire, moral judgment, or political power.* The things so ordered are integral parts of everyday life; indeed, they are among the most important things in our lives, impinging on religion, law, economics, and politics yet independent of them.

Under a gold monetary standard, unlike under a fiat paper "legal tender" standard, the state cannot create money by means of printing presses and by defining the product as the only legal form of currency. From the time of the French Revolution until the outbreak of World War I, the gold standard was regarded as an indispensable element of the principle of limited government. The gold standard, perhaps even more than a parliamentary system or federalism and a system of checks and balances—symbolized that the powers of the government were not only strictly limited, but that the state respected that limitation.

The difference between the lesion standard of disease and the fiat standard of (mental) illness is similar to the difference between the gold monetary standard and the fiat-paper-money standard. The Virchowian standard is fixed by biological-physical criteria, limiting the medical system from arbitrarily expanding its scope and hence its power. Neither doctors, patients, politicians, nor any other interested parties can create diseases by manipulating the language. *New diseases cannot be invented; they have to be discovered.* In contrast, the psychopathological standard of disease is flexible, letting medical and political authorities and popular opinion define, ad hoc, what should or should not count as a disease; they do so by attaching diagnostic labels to unwanted behaviors.

Between approximately 1850 and 1914, the Virchowian standard of disease and the gold standard of money were widely accepted as indispensable elements of scientific medical practice and sound economic policy: they provided the social context for the development of medical science and the growth of liberal democracies based on individual liberty, the right to property, and free markets.

The maintenance of scientific standards depends on agreement and authority, whereas the maintenance of moral and legal standards depends on tradition and power. Defining disease (and treatment) has long been the privilege of physicians. Today, it is largely the privilege of the therapeutic state.[3] To be sure, people in all walks of life have the "right" to call anything they wish a disease (or a treatment). However, once they act on that premise, they may be breaking the law—for example, the drug laws.

Let us call things by their proper names. Medical practice is a government monopoly, not a science. Only persons licensed by the state can call themselves "physicians" and only they are permitted to perform the healing acts the state defines as medical practice. In their relations to patients, physicians must follow strict rules and regulations, called "standards of practice," and are permitted to prescribe to their patients only substances that the state defines as legal drugs. Deviations from these rules are criminal offenses punished with harsh penalties. I suggested calling this arrangement "mono-medicine."[4] Like monogamy and monotheism, monomedicine is imposed by the state and taken for granted as "naturally right" by the people. In *1984,* slavery was called "freedom." Today, the state monopoly of medicine is called "private medical practice" and "medical freedom."

Monetary and disease standards affect people's everyday lives more directly and more pervasively than do scientific standards. There is no need here to retell the checkered history of monetary standards based on precious metals.[5] Suffice it to note that the practice of debasing the value of currency by minting coins containing decreased quantities of precious metals and increased quantities of base metals is thousands of years old. Paper money lends itself perfectly to creating monetary value out of an inexpensive product, paper. In his classic, *The Economic Consequences of the Peace,* John Maynard Keynes observed, "Lenin was certainly right. There is no subtler, no surer means of overturning the existing basis of society than to debauch the currency. The process engages all the hidden forces of economic law on the side of destruction, and does it in a manner which not one man in a million is able to diagnose."[6]

In *Pharmacracy: Medicine and Politics in America,* I showed that long before Virchow formulated a precise pathological standard of disease, that standard was subverted by a *diagnostic* inflation, fueled especially by the needs of the eighteenth-century medical specialty called "mad-doctoring." I say *subverted* because the pioneer nineteenth-century psychiatrists did not create a separate nonpathological standard of disease. On the contrary, they emphasized their professional identity as scientific physicians by adhering to a strict Virchowian lesion standard of disease: they regarded neurology and psychiatry as closely allied medical specialties, viewed themselves as neuro-psychiatrists, and attached medical-sounding labels ("diagnoses") to certain behaviors, exemplified by masturbation and homosexuality. Then, conflating diagnoses with diseases, they claimed to have discovered new brain diseases. In fact, they did no such thing. Instead, they medicalized human problems traditionally perceived in religious terms, transforming sins and crimes—such as self-murder, self-abuse, and self-medication—into sicknesses.

I V

Rudolf Virchow did not create the pathological standard of disease out of thin air. His achievement lay in concisely reformulating a concept and a criterion that had been developing for more than a century. Medical historian Roy Porter states, "This eagerness to ascribe madness to the body was most systematically codified in the teachings of Herman Boerhaave, the highly influential Leiden medical professor."[7] Boerhaave (1668–1738), famed Dutch physician, anatomist, botanist, chemist, and humanist, "insisted on the postmortem examination of patients whereby he demonstrated the relation of symptoms to lesions."[8] Boerhaave, a true pioneer of scientific medicine, committed himself to the premise that madness was a disease, and that disease was, by definition, a lesion located in the body.

In short, the view that madness is a bodily disease was a postulate or premise, nothing more. It seemed scientific but had nothing to do with science. Instead, it expressed the "enlightened" revolt against religious explanations of nature and the prevailing humanist-positivist Zeitgeist. In this spirit, Pierre Jean Georges Cabanis (1757–1808), a famed French physician and fervent Jacobin, declared, "The brain secretes thought as the liver secretes bile." Dutch physiologist Jakob Moleschott (1822–1893) gave the idea a renal twist, "The brain secretes thought as the kidney secretes urine."[9]

It is the doctrinal belief of contemporary biologists, neuroscientists, neurophilosophers, and psychiatrists that mind is brain and vice versa. Daniel C. Dennett, professor of philosophy at Tufts University, declares, "The mind is the brain."[10] Alan J. Hobson, professor of psychiatry at Harvard, explains, "[T]he brain and mind are one. . . . They are one entity. . . . I use the hyphenated term 'brain-mind' to denote unity."[11] Nobel laureate celebrity biologist Christian de Duve writes, "Mind is in the head, sustained by the brain. . . . The two are indissolubly linked, leading to the notion that thoughts, feelings, and all other manifestations of the mind are products of the activities of the brain. The concept is not new. The same was said two centuries ago."[12]

De Duve's writings are a mixture of Catholic apologetics and collectivist-positivist denial of individual responsibility. He approvingly cites the

Church's approval of evolution: "It has already been mentioned that the Catholic Church, long opposed to the notion of evolution, has recently bowed before the evidence of facts,"[13] as if that endorsement added to Darwinism's explanatory power. Then he adds some conceited lucubrations: "Moral responsibilities and ethical concerns likewise have become globalized, in areas such as environmental protection or bioethical safeguards, for example World organizations and world congresses abound. So it appears that the humankind has become a *supraorganism,* composed of multiple organs kept together by a growing network of integrative communications."[14] After citing Cabanis and Moleschott's assertions that the mind is "secreted" by the brain, de Duve concludes, "How could they be faulted? The proofs are there, indisputable."[15]

Proofs of what? That the mind is secreted by the brain just as bile and urine are secreted by liver and kidney? That is patent nonsense. Psychiatrists call manic depression and schizophrenia, the paradigmatic mental illnesses, "mood disorders" and "thought disorders." Thought and mood, unlike bile or urine, are not material things. Psychiatrists cannot observe them directly. Instead, they infer the subject's "mood disorder" and "thought disorder" from observations of his behavior, especially verbal and social behavior. Samuel H. Barondes, professor and director of the Center for Neurobiology and Psychiatry at the University of California at San Francisco, acknowledges that he does not want to be bound by a materialist definition of (mental) illness. He writes:

> Since the primary concern of this article is mental illness, it is critical that we agree at the outset that such illness does exist. Although this proposition may seem self-evident, it remains a source of confusion or debate (Szasz, 1961). There is, for example, a reluctance to call someone mentally ill, inasmuch as the border between illness and normality is not well defined. There is also disagreement about whether "normal" means average or ideal. *What is clear, however, is that there are patterns of behavior that are very uncomfortable for a person and for those with whom he or she interacts. And some patterns are so maladaptive that illness is obviously a proper designation.*[16]

Behavior is "real," but it is not a material "thing." Manic depression and schizophrenia qua mood and thought disorders do not belong in the same

DEFINING DISEASE | *49*

table of diseases as hepatitis and uremia qua liver and kidney disorders. If we use mental illness terms as the names of brain diseases, as many physicians do, then they belong in a table of diseases with multiple sclerosis and stroke, not in a table with pedophilia and pyromania.

v

Healing the body (medicine) and healing the soul (religion) are established social institutions, sanctioned by custom and law. Persons are not disembodied objects; they are, literally, embodied or incarnated beings. *Webster's* defines the verb "to embody" as "to become material" and defines "incarnate" as "to make flesh." When religion reigned, the devil was incarnated in the serpent or in persons called "possessed." Christianity incarnated God in the body of a man called "Jesus." When medicine replaced religion as the dominant institution concerned with bodily healing (and left spiritual healing to religion), madness was reincarnated as bodily disease. This metamorphosis is clearly displayed in the writings of Benjamin Rush (1746–1813), the "father" of American psychiatry.

Rush was no mere practitioner of medicine. He was a man of the Enlightenment, a physician who fancied himself a scientist. He did not know what ailed the mad persons who were entrusted to his care. As a "scientific" physician, he *assumed* that all his patients—in fact, masses of people who were not his or anyone else's patients—had a bodily disease. His following assertions are illustrative: "Lying is a corporeal disease. . . . Suicide is madness."[17]

Pathological changes in the body, especially in the nervous system, cause abnormal behaviors. Therefore, it is not unreasonable to assume that abnormal behaviors are due to pathological changes in the body. As we know, medical research has lent some support to this assumption—for example, in cases where "mental disorders" can be shown to be the consequences of infections, metabolic disorders, or nutritional deficiencies.

However, the criteria for what behaviors count as abnormal are cultural, ethical, religious, and legal, not medical or scientific. Therefore, it is a priori absurd to try to explain all abnormal behaviors by attributing them to brain diseases. The dilemma thus posed was overcome by creating the concept of psychopathology, a category of illnesses with (metaphorical) "mental lesions." While the late-nineteenth-century pathologists and bacteriologists were busy discovering and describing new somatic pathologies, psychiatrists were busy "discovering" and describing new psychopathologies, each ostensibly a disease of the central nervous system.

One of the most important practitioners in the art of manufacturing mental diseases was Baron Richard von Krafft-Ebing (1840–1902), a German-born psychiatrist who was professor of psychiatry, successively, at the Universities of Strasbourg, Graz, and Vienna. The work that made Krafft-Ebing world famous is *Psychopathia Sexualis,* the first edition of which appeared in 1886. Krafft-Ebing was an early practitioner of transforming, with the aid of Latin and a medical diploma, behaviors considered sinful into sicknesses. Psychiatrists authoritatively classified *sexual perversions* as "cerebral neuroses" and lawyers, politicians, and the public eagerly embraced the reality of the new diseases: thus did modern sexology become an integral part of medicine and the new science of psychiatry.[18] Sigmund Freud extended Krafft-Ebing's pathologizing of behavior from sexual behavior to everyday behavior. Although Freud viewed "neuroses" as motivated behaviors, he insisted that they nonetheless were bona fide diseases.[19]

Today, the most self-referential and naive mistaking of a metaphor for the thing metaphorized is regarded as a medical discovery. Alvin Poussaint, professor of psychiatry at Harvard Medical School, declares, "My position is that extreme racism is a serious mental illness because it represents a delusional disorder."[20]

Frank Tallis, a British psychologist who teaches neuroscience at the Institute of Psychiatry at King's College in London and is the author of *Love Sick: Love as a Mental Illness,* explains, "Lovesickness can even be lethal, as when rejection and unrequited love increase the risk of suicide. . . . Studies suggest that when people fall in love and begin to obsess, it causes a drop in the level of serotonin, a brain chemical. . . . Medication also might be helpful."[21]

Other love researchers report, "The [magnetic resonance] scanning shows that love activates specific regions in the reward system of the brain, while reducing activity in the systems involved in making negative judgments. . . . [T]he most activated parts of the brain were those which respond to oxytocin and vasopressin."[22]

Psychiatric explanations of so-called abnormal behaviors ought to alert us to pay more attention to what we regard as an explanation. Does calling transubstantiation a miracle explain it? Does calling pedophilia a mental illness explain it? Perhaps our very concept of explanation, framed in ordinary language, is biased by our deep-seated conceits and fashionable preconceptions. The Hungarian term for explanation suggests that such, indeed, may often be the case.

The Hungarian word for "Hungarian" is *magyar*. The same term serves as the root for "explanation," which is *magyarázat;* "to explain" is *megmagyaráz;* "inexplicable" is *megmagyarázhatatlan,* literally, "it cannot be said in Hungarian"; and the command to say something clearly is *mond (beszélj) magyarul,* that is, "say it in Hungarian." Hungarians are not aware that their term for explanation and therefore their concept of it are so linguistically self-centered. Perhaps one has to change cultures and retain an interest in the idiosyncrasies of one's mother tongue to appreciate such a semantic oddity.

For Hungarians, then, an explanation of anything is "saying it in Hungarian," as if saying it—whatever "it" may be—in another language were incomprehensible, lacking the essential element of explanation. For us today, the explanation of a behavior is saying it in the language of mental illness, brain, dopamine, and drugs. Saying it in plain English is not scientific, not explanatory, not "true."

VI

Medical scientists need a gold standard of disease—a clear, objective demarcation between disease and nondisease. Practicing physicians, patients, politicians, and the public want a fiat standard of disease, unconstrained by objective criteria, a demarcation between disease and nondisease open to change in accordance with fluctuating economic, ideological, and political interests and fashions. As a result we have, in effect, two tables of diseases: one contains only somatic pathological entities; the other is composed of a mixture of such entities together with a host of human conditions unrelated to somatic pathology. The two systems are mutually parasitic. Elastic criteria of disease make it easier for medical scientists to obtain ideological and economic support from government and private industry, but imperil their scientific integrity; physicians, patients, politicians, and the public gain the imprimatur of science for satisfying their economic and existential interests by means of pseudomedical methods, but lose their ability to think clearly about illness and treatment.

The phrase *laissez faire, laissez passer* (let things alone, let them pass) was coined by the eighteenth-century French physiocrats as an injunction against government interference with trade. The first half of the phrase became the slogan of free market economists. Although the term *laissez faire,* usually hyphenated, is now a part of the English language, its practice—especially in medicine—has become passé. Every modern state is a dirigiste therapeutic state. Today, medicine is an integral part of the modern political economy; indeed, it is the single most important part. Modern psychiatry is a branch of the law, family court, and criminal justice system rather than a branch of medicine. Scientific criteria of disease are confined to the pages of journals and textbooks of general pathology and the pathologies of various organ systems—for example, dermatopathology and neuropathology.

Not surprisingly, the modern medical expert, especially if he is also an expert on philosophy and medical ethics, is contemptuous of the gold standard of disease, or indeed of any standard of it. Rejecting the desirability of a boundary between disease and nondisease has become the very hallmark of the contemporary "progressive" medical philosopher. Germund Hesslow, professor of neuroscience and associate professor of philosophy at Lund University in Sweden, asks, "Do we need a concept of disease?" and answers, "The health/disease question is irrelevant—*we do not really have to know whether someone has a disease or not, and consequently we do not need a definition of 'disease.'"*[23] That declaration might well serve as the manifesto of pharmacracy and the therapeutic state.

The old quacks peddled fake cures to treat real diseases. The new quacks peddle fake diseases to justify chemical pacification and medical coercion. The old quacks were politically harmless: they could harm individuals only with those individuals' consent. The new quacks are a serious threat to individual liberty and personal responsibility: they are agents of the therapeutic state who can and do harm individuals both with and without those individuals' consent. Theocracy is the alliance of religion with the state. Pharmacracy is the alliance of medicine with the state.

PART TWO

Disturbing Behavior and Medicine's Responses to It

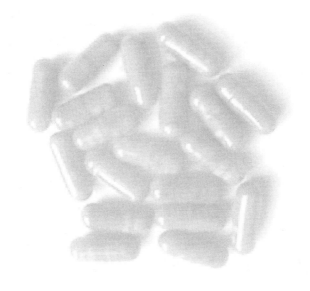

8

The Origin of Psychiatry

Coercion as Cure

Sir Roderick Glossop . . . is always called a nerve specialist, because it sounds better, but everybody knows that he's really a sort of janitor to the looney-bin.

—P. G. Wodehouse, *The Inimitable Jeeves* (1923)

I

AT THE BEGINNING of the seventeenth century, there were no mental hospitals, as we now know them. To be sure, there were a few facilities— such as Bethlehem Hospital, better known as Bedlam—in which a small number, usually less than a dozen, of pauper insane were confined. By the end of the century, however, there was a flourishing new industry, called the "trade in lunacy."[1]

To understand the modern concept of mental illness, one must focus on the radically different origins of the medical and psychiatric professions. Medicine began with sick persons seeking relief from their suffering. Psychiatry began with the relatives of unwanted, troublesome persons seeking relief from the embarrassment and suffering their kin caused them. Unlike the regular doctor, the early psychiatrist, called mad-doctor, treated persons who did not want to be his patients, and whose ailments manifested themselves by exciting the resentment of their relatives. These are critical issues never to be lost sight of.

Annoying, unconventional behavior must have existed for as long as human beings have lived together in society. Psychiatry begins when people stop interpreting such behavior in religious and existential terms and begin to interpret it in medical terms. The fatal weakness of most psychiatric historiographies lies in the historians' failure to give sufficient weight to the role of coercion in psychiatry and to acknowledge that mad-doctoring had nothing to do with healing.

II

Higher mammals, especially humans, remain dependent on their parents for some time after birth. Because only women can bear children and because caring for infants is a time-consuming job, societies have adopted the familiar gender-based job differentiation, females caring for the young and tending the shelter, males providing food and protection for the family.

Once a society advances beyond the stage of subsistence economy, mother surrogates often replace the nurturing role of the biological mother. For centuries, parents who could afford household help delegated the task of child care to servants—governesses for infants and young children, tutors for older ones.

The belief that all parents passionately love their children and would like nothing better than be able to take care of them is a modern fiction and self-delusion. Taking care of children, day in and day out, is not a very interesting activity. Many adults dislike being merely in the company of a small child. Most people feel similarly disinclined to care for an insane adult, that is, for a person who is selfish and self-absorbed, demanding and dependent, intemperately happy or unhappy, perhaps even threatening and violent. Stripped of three hundred years of psychiatric-semantic embellishments, the fact is that a mad person appears to relatives as an unpleasant individual whose company they would rather avoid. Burdened by such an unwanted individual, they use psychiatric "care" to dispose of their family member.

Mad adults are, however, not children. Children have neither the physical strength nor the political power to resist being controlled by their parents and their deputies who possess lawful authority over them. The adult does. Other adults, whether parents or siblings, have no rights over their adult relatives, provided they are sane. Before adults can be treated as a mad, they must first be divested of their rights.[2] Reframing the political status of the insane adult as similar to that of a child needing care accomplishes this task.

III

Historically, psychiatry's first order of business was to establish insanity as a genuine disease, that is, as neither malingering nor an (immoral or illegal) act carried out by a responsible adult. Its next business was to distinguish insanity from other diseases and assign to it the singular characteristic of having the power to deprive the patient of his higher mental faculties, rendering him childlike, and justifying controlling and caring for him against his will. Hence the close association between severe head injury, brain disease (neurosyphilis), and insanity. This whole package was required by the political character of seventeenth-century English society, where, for the first time in history, a people dedicated themselves to honoring the values of liberty and property. It is not by accident that the ideas of limited government, the rule of law, and insanity as an infantilizing illness all arose and developed in England. Both the medicalization of madness and the infantilization of the insane were, and are, needed to reconcile a society's devotion to the ideals of individual liberty and responsibility with its desire to relieve itself of certain troublesome individuals by means other than those provided by the criminal law.

The idea of insanity as a condition requiring the mad-housing of the insane was invented by those who needed it, the members of the dominant classes of seventeenth-century English society. It was they who had to carry the burden of being responsible for their mad relatives by having to provide for their needs and who, at the same time, had to conform their behavior to the requirements of a social order that placed a high value on the liberty of persons and the ownership of property. What was a man to do with his spouse, adult child, or elderly parent who flaunted convention and perhaps neglected his own health, but who was considered to possess a basic right to liberty and property? The time was past when such a troublesome individual could be treated as a clan member, responsible to the group, devoid of individual rights in the modern sense. The rule of law liquidated the autocratic prerogatives of elders vis-à-vis deviant adults. From the seventeenth century onward, the adult members of families were held together more by cooperation and compromise, and less or not at all by direct coercion. Regrettably, cooperation and compromise are useless vis-à-vis persons who are unable or unwilling to cooperate and compromise.

These political and legal developments placed family members faced with a disturbing relative in a difficult situation. Though embarrassed and victimized by their (mad) kinfolk, the (sane) relatives could not control their relative by means of the informal, interpersonal mechanisms normally used to harmonize relations in the family. They had only two options, both useless. One was to set the engine of the criminal law against offending family members (provided they had broken the law), a course that would have led to the social or physical death of the mad relative and the abject humiliation of the family. The other was to expel them from their homes, a course that would have required the sane relatives to possess more power than those they wanted to expel and would therefore have been most impractical when it was (felt to be) most necessary. It was an intolerable impasse. Sane (or perhaps merely scheming) family members had to come up with a socially acceptable arrangement to enable them to control, by means of a noncriminal legal procedure, the unwanted adult relative (who was senile, incompetent, troublesome, or perhaps simply in the way). That was the need that generated the concept of mental illness, and that is the reason why the concept of mental illness differs so radically from the concept of bodily illness. The point is that the physically ill person can be cared for without requiring coercive social control, but the so-called mentally ill person cannot be cared for in this way because he or she (rightly) rejects the patient role.

In what way did a property-owning madman in England in, say, 1650 endanger his relatives? He did so in one or all of the following ways: personally, by embarrassing them; economically, by dissipating his assets; and physically, by attacking his relatives. In this connection, it is necessary to acknowledge that a person who spurns our core values—that life, liberty, and property are goods worth preserving—endangers not only himself and his relatives but, symbolically, society and the social fabric itself. The madman's embarrassing behavior gave his family impetus for hiding him; his improvidence, which provided an important conceptual bridge between the old notion of incompetence and the new idea of insanity, gave them an impetus for dealing with him as if he were incompetent. The law had long recognized mental retardation as a justification for placing the mentally deficient person under guardianship. Now the law was asked to do the same for the mentally deranged person. Medieval English guardianship procedures lent powerful support to the emerging practice of madhousing. Both procedures grew from the soil of English political-economic and legal tradition, grounded in the value of preserving landed wealth and ensuring its stable transmission in the family. As far back as the thirteenth century, common law recognized two classes of incompetents: idiots, mentally subnormal from birth, who were considered to be permanently impaired; and lunatics, normal persons who went mad, who were considered to be capable of recovery. The procedure for declaring a person a lunatic was similar to that of declaring him incompetent: "Commissions examined such persons before a jury that ruled on their sanity. . . . Physicians played essentially no role in the certification process itself."[3]

Long before pauper lunatics were exiled to madhouses, propertied persons considered to be mad were managed in a manner that presaged the practice of mad-doctoring: "Physical supervision and care of the disabled party was commonly handled by retaining a live-in servant, the so-called 'lunatics keeper,' a person usually of the same gender as the disabled individual. . . . Boarding out the lunatic or idiot at a private dwelling, in the company of a servant, was also commonplace; this practice in some respects anticipated the development of private madhouses in the eighteenth century."[4]

IV

Although some special facilities for housing lunatics existed before the seventeenth century—for example, in ancient Greece, in medieval England, and in Islamic societies—these were isolated arrangements for looking after a few unwanted individuals. They were not instances of an institutional arrangement serving the explicit purpose of incarcerating persons categorized as insane. The history of mental hospitalization, as we know it, began in seventeenth-century England, when and where, for the first time in history, the care of the insane was systematically delegated to persons outside the family. Forcibly removed from home, the mad person was forcibly rehoused in the home of a surrogate caretaker.

Who wants to deprive us of life, liberty, and property? Enemies abroad, criminals at home, and the state to which we entrust the power to protect us from them. These threats are external to our selves. Our lives, liberties, and properties may also be threatened, metaphorically speaking, from within, by the self acting in opposition to interests attributed to it by others. In fact, *the metaphor of the self divided against itself is as central to psychiatry as the metaphor of the Trinity is to Christianity*. The "split personality" of schizophrenia is only the most familiar example. Psychiatrists have managed to infect the Western mind with many other examples of "divided selves," such as the true versus the false self, the authentic versus the inauthentic self, the sane or healthy versus the insane or sick self, and so forth. To be sure, we all harbor diverse desires, some at odds with others, but we have only one self per person. The force of the maxim "Actions speak louder than words" lies largely in its power to prevent the disuniting of actor and action. However, it is precisely the lying truth of that separation that we legitimize when we assert that a person who neglects himself or his property or who harms or kills himself is "not himself." People have always engaged in such behaviors. In religious societies, they were viewed as martyrs, sinners, or persons possessed by demons. In the West since the Enlightenment, they have been viewed as mentally ill.

To see through the confusions embodied in the image of the mentally ill person as "not himself," we must be clear about the connection between behavior and disease. Every part of our body influences our behavior. If we have arthritis, we cannot move normally. If we have glaucoma, we cannot see normally. The organ affecting behavior most directly is the brain. If it is seriously damaged, we die; if less seriously damaged, we lose a wide range of bodily functions, such as the ability to see or speak. The question we must keep in mind is: when and why do we attribute a person's behavior to brain disease, and when and why do we not do so? Briefly, the answer is that we often attribute bad behavior to disease (to excuse the agent), never attribute good behavior to disease (lest we deprive the agent of credit), and typically attribute good behavior to free will and insist that bad behavior called mental illness is a "no fault" act of nature.[5]

v

There is a sound medical basis for the disease model of derangement, namely, the illness now known as neurosyphilis or paresis. In seventeenth-century

England, syphilis caused many people to become mad. But many mad people did not have syphilis. The paucity of medical knowledge at the time made it virtually impossible for people to know whether a particular person's abnormal behavior was or was not due to brain disease. However, even then, there was a simple and reliable method for distinguishing persons whose brains were being destroyed by syphilis from those who went mad for other reasons. The syphilitic madmen died, usually within a year or two after admission to hospital, whereas the healthy madmen often outlived their sane mad-doctors.

Although a person may behave abnormally because of having a brain disease, the typical madman behaves the way he does because of his particular adaptation to the events that comprise his life. Examples abound in Shakespeare's tragedies. King Lear goes mad because of his poor choice for retirement. Lady Macbeth is driven mad by guilt and remorse over a criminal career. Hamlet breaks down under the stress of discovering that his mother and uncle murdered his father. Yet none of these persons is relocated in a madhouse. Why? Because there are no madhouses. A century later, the practice of resolving such family conflicts by letting the stronger party psychiatrically dispose of the weaker one was well on its way of becoming accepted in principle, established in practice, ratified by law, and embraced by the public.

Some people have always found it difficult to grow up and assume the responsibilities of adulthood. Formerly, the person who failed to meet this universal challenge—who remained unskilled, unmarried, unemployed, and unemployable—was cared for in the family or became a vagrant, leading a marginal existence. His relatives, if they were educated and had a large vocabulary, might have called him a "tatterdemalion." Now they call him "schizophrenic." Regardless of such a person's medical condition, there is a clear and critical connection between the value we attach to life, liberty, and property and the idea of insanity. The "misbehavior" of a prostate is not a moral issue, but the misbehavior of a person is. The distinction is useful for the observer-respondent: if he accepts the moral dimension of insanity, he is faced with an ethical-political problem, whereas if he rejects it, he is faced with a medical-technical problem.

Of course, there is rationale, though not validity, in bracketing the insane with infants. There are similarities between the behavior of an adult who does not eat or sleep properly, neglects possessions, perhaps even attacks relatives, and the behavior of an unruly child.[6] That analogy is the basis for the legal-psychological strategy of treating insane persons as if they were (like) infants. Correlatively, the relatives of a misbehaving (mad) adult feel compelled to protect their relative as well as themselves from embarrassing and destructive behavior. The legal-psychological strategy is to let psychiatrists act as guardians of their patients and treat them as if they were (like) children.

At the beginning of the trade in lunacy, the individuals incarcerated as insane were members of the propertied classes who posed a problem to their families. The sane relatives' problem was not finding a home for a homeless person, but finding a justification for removing the lawful occupant of a home from his residence and relocating him in someone else's home. Although the historical record is clear, Michel Foucault constructed a history of psychiatry that has confused the matter. Influenced by his Marxist bias, he traced the origin of the practice of incarcerating madmen to the segregation of lepers and, more specifically, to the large-scale confinement of urban indigents in France in the seventeenth century.[7] Although some of what Foucault described did happen, it was not the way the systematic confinement of persons diagnosed as mad came into being. Individual rights were virtually nonexistent in seventeenth-century France. They were assuredly nonexistent for the propertyless French masses. Hence, imprisoning the rabble in "general hospitals" did not require the pretext of insanity as an illness. It is simply not true that institutional psychiatry represented the beginning of a new mode of warfare between the haves and have-nots, the former resorting to the tactic of labeling the latter as insane in order to remove them to the madhouse. The incarceration of rich persons in private madhouses came first and was followed, considerably later, by the incarceration of poor persons in public insane asylums. Roy Porter emphasizes that psychiatry was *not* "a discipline for controlling the rabble. . . . Provision of public asylums did not become mandatory until 1845. . . . Even at the close of the eighteenth century, the tally of the confined mad poor in Bristol, a town of some 30,000, was only twenty. . . . [Whereas] about 400 people a year were being admitted to private asylums."[8]

VI

Except for some historians of psychiatry, few people today realize that the early madhouses were *not hospitals* in the modern sense of that term. They were simply the keepers' homes into which they took a few, often only one or two, madmen or madwomen as involuntary boarders or houseguests. The keepers, who owned and operated these private madhouses, were laypeople, principally clergymen, pointing to an important connection between religion (the cure of souls) and mad-doctoring (the cure of minds).

The practice of healing began as an undifferentiated religious-medical enterprise. At a much later stage of history, as the social world split into sacred and profane parts, the practice of healing also split: one part remained a religious activity, the other part became the profession of medicine. In the West, this separation occurred twice: first, with respect to the body, in Greece, two and a half millennia ago; second, with respect to the mind, in England, less than four hundred years ago. Since the Enlightenment, spiritual and scientific healing have become, and have been perceived as, distinct and separate enterprises.

There is a long Western tradition of interpreting insanity in religious terms; treating it as due to demonic possession, by means of exorcism; and, most importantly, viewing clerical coercion as morally laudable and politically legitimate. When people believed that eternal life in the hereafter was more important than a brief sojourn on earth, torturing the possessed person to improve the quality of his life after death was regarded as an act of beneficence. Therefore the long history of lawful clerical coercion.

In contrast, before the seventeenth century, there was no tradition justifying the use of force by physicians. Unlike the doctor of divinity, the doctor of medicine had no right (yet) to imprison and torture his patients. In fact, when Englishmen first tried to enlist the doctor in the service of diagnosing and disposing their problematic relatives, the physician, as Shakespeare described in Macbeth, declined the invitation. This rejection was consistent with the physician's historical mandate. From ancient times, his help was sought by suffering persons on their own behalf, or by healthy persons on behalf of relatives too disabled to seek help for themselves. The clergyman labored under no such tradition, which explains his role as pioneer mad-doctor and madhouse keeper. Subsequently, as the clergyman's power diminished, the mad-doctor's increased, and theological coercion was replaced by psychiatric coercion.

The trade in lunatics must be understood primarily in existential-economic terms. The enterprise satisfied the existential needs of the lunatics' relatives, and the economic needs of the entrepreneurs who provided a service for which there was a market.

The madhouse keeper's customers were persons of means, able and willing to pay to relieve them of the company of their unwanted relative. The keepers were relatively impecunious, eager to please their customers. Contemporary observers recognized the essentially commercial character of the transaction. Thomas Bakewell, himself the proprietor of a madhouse, observed, "The pecuniary interest of the proprietor and the secret wishes of the lunatics' relatives, led not only to the neglect of all means of cure, but also to the prevention and delay of recovery."[9] Another madhouse keeper wrote, "If a man comes in here mad, we'll keep him so; if he is in his senses, we'll soon drive him out of them."[10] The practice of involuntary mental hospitalization or psychiatric slavery thus began as a private, capitalist enterprise. Like chattel slavery, it too had to be sanctioned and enforced by the state.

Because madhousing was soon transformed into a largely statist program of confining troublesome poor people, the entrepreneurial origin of psychiatry as a form of private imprisonment merits reemphasis. In the seventeenth century, England was essentially a two-class society, divided between propertied and propertyless persons. Because property, especially in land, generated income, members of the upper classes did not have to work to procure a livelihood for themselves and their families. The unpropertied, whose only property was their labor, had to work or face destitution. Therefore, their relatives had nothing to gain, and much to lose, by having them declared mad. The very propertylessness of the poor thus protected them from the greed of their relatives and the depredations of the mad-doctors who catered to them.

Ironically, long before the misery of poorly paid factory workers generated denunciations of private profit, the early critics of madhouses blamed the abuses of the trade in lunacy on the profit motive. It was, to be sure, an important factor, but it was merely a symptom. Forbes B. Winslow, the proprietor of two private asylums, denounced the practice of patients being "brought into the market and offered for sale, like a flock of sheep, to the highest bidder."[11] He was referring to the madhouse keepers' practice of advertising for "guests." A typical advertisement ran as follows: "Insanity. Twenty per cent. annually on the receipts will be guaranteed to any medical man recommending a quiet patient of either sex, to a first class asylum, with highest testimonials."[12] Plus ça change . . . Today, private mental hospitals not only advertise their services but encourage their staff to double as psychiatric bounty hunters. It hardly needs adding that the madhouse keepers hawk their wares not to the so-called patients but to their relatives who are eager to get rid of them. Since government and insurance programs now pick up the tab, this tactic has become more popular than ever.

Unfortunately, the early critics of the madhouse business aimed their fire at the wrong target. The root problem was not profit but power, the mad-doctor's power to lawfully transform a sovereign British subject from a person with a right to liberty into a mental patient deprived of that right. How and why did this happen when it happened and where it happened? The short answer is, because of the particular economic-political conditions in late-seventeenth-century England: the trade in lunacy—that is to say, the business of private mad-doctoring—the free market, limited government, and the debtor's prison were all English inventions; ironically, each was a consequence of the spread of commerce, capitalism, and individualism, that is, individual liberty and personal responsibility. The writings of seventeenth- and eighteenth-century English physicians, calling mental illness an "English malady," support this interpretation.

Morbus Anglicus, a treatise by Gideon Harvey, physician to King Charles II, appeared in 1672. The ailment he had in mind was "hypochondriacal melancholy."[13] In 1733, George Cheyne popularized Harvey's idea in his classic work by the same title in English, *The English Malady.* This book remains of interest and importance because it exemplifies the confusion between metaphorical maladies of the soul and literal diseases of the body, a confusion that continues to characterize psychiatry today.[14] "The Spirit of a Man," wrote Cheyne, "can bear his Infirmities, but a wounded Spirit who can bear? saith a Prophet. As this is a great Truth in the Intellectual World, so it may allude to the Human machine."[15] To what conditions did Cheyne refer when he categorized them as instances of the "English Malady"? They were "Spleen," "Vapours," "Lowness of Spirits," "Hysterical Distemper," and other similar ailments. Despite naming "it" "Lowness of Spirits," he identified the condition as a bodily disease and recommended treating it with mercury, antimony, and other arcane compounds and concoctions, as well as dietary regimens and purgatives.[16]

Old confusion? No, new "science": In our day, certain human difficulties are, by fiat, "brain diseases." The "Jerusalem Syndrome," "Stockholm Syndrome," "Oslo Syndrome," and "Paris Syndrome" are all specific "diseases" identified and named by psychiatrists and listed on Web sites.[17] Einstein was right: "Only two things are infinite, the universe and human stupidity, and I'm not sure about the former."

VII

Every solution to a human problem generates a new set of problems. Madhousing the unwanted family member was a novel method for coping with an old familial and social problem. Inevitably, protest against a novel social practice arises in the same cultural milieu as does the "reform." The Industrial Revolution and the Luddite revolt against the machine both began in England about the same time. And so did psychiatric slavery and the protests against it.

Insofar as insanity is accepted as a justification for depriving a person of liberty, the basic risk inherent in involuntary mental hospitalization becomes analogous to the risk inherent in imprisoning criminals: a person might be wrongfully identified, as insane or guilty of a crime, and wrongfully deprived of liberty. Preoccupation with the wrongful confinement of sane persons in insane asylums, called "false commitment," is a leitmotif that runs through the entire history of psychiatry, to this very day. It is a chronicle of protest on the part of the allegedly falsely committed person proclaiming his sanity, while acknowledging the insanity of his fellow victims and applauding their incarceration as just and proper. It seemed not to occur to the protestors to challenge the legitimacy of psychiatric slavery itself. Mad and sane alike accepted the principle that the illness called insanity justifies incarcerating the patient.[18]

Fortunately, madmen and madwomen claiming to be sane were not the only critics of the madhouse system. Their impeached voices were amplified and supported by the unimpeachable reports of journalists and men of letters. These critics alerted the public to the fact that individuals were often committed not because they needed care but because they were the victims of scheming relatives and greedy madhouse keepers. These accusations were supported by anecdotes of philandering husbands committing their innocent wives and greedy children confining their harmless elderly parents. Obsession with false commitment thus obscured the fundamental issue of the freedom and responsibility of the so-called mad person, and reinforced the belief that incarcerating the truly insane was in the best interests of both the patient and society. One example must suffice.

Daniel Defoe (1660–1731), the author of *Robinson Crusoe,* was what we would now call an investigative journalist. He was also a pioneer critic of the business of mad-doctoring. Like other madhouse reformers, Defoe objected only to the confining of sane persons, an abuse he attributed partly to the selfishness of the relatives initiating the commitment process and partly to the rapacity of the madhouse keepers. He wrote:

> This leads me to exclaim against the vile Practice now so much in vogue among the better Sort, as they are called, but the worst sort in fact, namely, the sending their Wives to Mad-Houses at every Whim or Dislike, that they may be more secure and undisturb'd in their Debaucheries. . . . This is the height of Barbarity and Injustice in a Christian Country, it is a clandestine Inquisition, nay worse. . . . Is it not enough to make anyone mad to be suddenly clap'd up, stripp'd, whipp'd, ill fed, and worse us'd? To have no Reason assign'd for such Treatment, no Crime alledg'd or accusers to confront? . . . In my humble Opinion all private Mad-Houses should be suppress'd at once.[19]

Note that Defoe speaks only of the practice of locking up persons of "the better Sort," as he called members of the propertied class. The large-scale commitment of the poor in public madhouses lay still in the future. Because they never questioned the idea of mental illness or the legitimacy of incarcerating persons diagnosed as insane, the critics of false commitment accomplished less than nothing. By shaming the madhouse keepers and society into prettifying the psychiatric plantations, they preserved and strengthened the system of psychiatric slavery. Psychiatrists became more sophisticated, concealing incarceration as hospitalization and torture as treatment. After 1800, the persistence of psychiatric abuses is attributed to a succession of fashionable scapegoats, such as untrained or sadistic doctors, inadequate government funding, the severity of the patients' diseases, the inadequacy of available treatments, and, today, to the overuse or underuse of psychiatric drugs.

VIII

During the eighteenth century, the English people were as engrossed with the idea of madness as the "abuse of reason" as we are with the idea of addiction as the "abuse of drugs." I have remarked elsewhere on some of the cultural and economic reasons for this development.[20] Among these, one of the most interesting and perceptive is Michael DePorte's attribution of the increasing interest in insanity to the policy at Bethlehem Hospital that began in the seventeenth century "of allowing visitors to come and go freely, a practice which not only gave writers a chance to observe madmen at first hand, but which also gave them an audience familiar with the behavior of the insane."[21] Visiting Bedlam as if it were a zoo not only gave artists a chance to observe madmen, it also gave madmen an opportunity to address a more sympathetic audience than their fellow victims and disdainful keepers.

Jonathan Swift (1667–1745) made many references to madness, mostly satirical. Like Shakespeare, he took for granted that there is method in it. In *A Tale of a Tub,* for example, he describes a madman as "a tailor run mad with pride,"[22] echoing Hobbes's interpretation of a half a century earlier: "The passion, whose violence, or continuance, maketh madness, is either great vainglory which is commonly called pride, and self-conceit; or great dejection of mind."[23] In the same essay, Swift ridicules the view that geniuses are insane and lashes out at sadistic practices that pass as mad-doctoring: "Epicurus, Diogenes, Appolonius, Lucretius, Paracelsus, Des Cartes, and others, who if they were now in the world . . . would in this our undistinguishing age incur manifest danger of phlebotomy, and whips, and chains, and dark chambers, and straw."[24] In his magisterial biography of Swift, Irvin Ehrenpreis writes,

"The theme of madness which runs through Swift's work normally carries the motif of power without responsibility. In Irish affairs it grows into the concept of a nation gone mad: Parliament as Bedlam populated by lunatics who think themselves statesmen, the kingdom as a land of absurdities . . . the machinery of government in Ireland has for its true function that of farcical entertainment, diverting people from their real problems."[25]

Swift views madness as a moral and political matter, not a medical malady. He uses the term "madness" as a figure of speech, an evocation of the turmoil and tragedy of human existence, not the diagnosis of a disease requiring medical intervention. Swift's conduct toward allegedly mad persons, himself included, was, however, inconsistent with his critical comments. He derided Bedlam as a place of "phlebotomy, whips, chain, dark chambers, and straw," yet joined the hospital's governing board and tried to commit one of his friends to it, who, Swift believed, "went mad from thinking too long about the problems of calculating longitude."[26] At the same time, he suggested that since "incurable fools, incurable rogues, incurable liars, [and] the incurably vain or envious" qualified for admission to Bethlehem Hospital, "a certificate as an 'incurable scribbler' would elect him [Swift] a patient at the foundation."[27]

The most powerful evidence of Swift's concern with madness is his last will, in which he bequeathed his estate for the construction of an insane asylum in Dublin, which as yet had none. His poem "Verses on the Death of Dr. Swift," written in 1732, ends with this grand double entendre:

He gave the little Wealth he had,
To build a House for Fools and Mad:
And shew'd by one satyric Touch,
No Nation wanted it so much.[28]

To his bequest of about eleven thousand pounds, a substantial sum at that time, other gifts were added, enabling the city in 1757, twelve years after Swift's death, to open St. Patrick's Hospital, better known as Swift's Hospital.

For Swift the immortal artist, madness was largely a metaphor for hypocrisy, perversity, and stupidity. However, for Swift the man who feared going mad, madness was a disease that might render the patient dangerous and hence justify his segregation. It must be recalled that during much of his adult life Swift suffered from Ménière's disease, or labyrinthine vertigo, which was then a mysterious ailment that made him fear for his own sanity.[29] In the poem in which he recorded his bequest, he described his condition thus:

> That old vertigo in his head
> Will never leave him till he's dead:
> Besides, his memory decays,
> He recollects not what he says;
> He cannot call his friends to mind;
> Forgets the place where he last din'd.[30]

Swift's fear of going mad suggests a sophisticated appreciation of the relationship between dementia as brain disease and the sorts of behaviors that were becoming characterized as manifestations of madness.

9

Hysteria as Language

"Then, to speak more plainly," continued the physician, . . . "hath all the operations of this disorder been fairly laid open and recounted to me?"

"How can you question it?" asked the minister [Mr. Dimmesdale]. "Surely it were child's play to call in a physician and then hide the sore!"

"You would tell me, then, that I know all? . . . He to whom only the outward and physical evil is laid open, knoweth, oftentimes, but half the evil which he is called upon to cure. A bodily disease, which we look upon as whole and entire within itself, may, after all, be but a symptom of some ailment in the spiritual part. . . .

"You deal not [said the clergyman], I take it, in medicine for the soul!" "Thus, a sickness," continued Roger Chillingworth, going on, in an unaltered tone, without heeding the interruption, . . . "a sickness, a sore place, if we may so call it, in your spirit hath immediately its appropriate manifestation in your bodily frame. Would you, therefore, that your physician heal the bodily evil? How may this be unless you first lay open to him the wound or trouble in your soul?"

"No, not to thee! not to an earthly physician!" cried Mr. Dimmesdale, . . . "Not to thee! But, if it be the soul's disease, then do I commit myself to the one Physician of the soul! . . . But who art thou, that meddlest in this matter? that dares thrust himself between the sufferer and his God?"

—Nathaniel Hawthorne,
The Scarlet Letter (1850)

I

HYSTERIA IS THE NAME PSYCHIATRISTS GIVE to a form of mental illness characterized by the display of bodily signs, such as paralysis or spasmodic movements, and by complaints about the body, such as lack of feeling or pain. Other terms for the phenomenon are "conversion hysteria" and "dissociative reaction." Bodily communications indistinguishable from those characteristic of hysteria may be presented also by individuals diagnosed as malingering, hypochondriacal, neurasthenic, or schizophrenic, and by so-called normal persons as well.

The phenomena we call "hysteria" and regard as a mental disease have been known since antiquity. Their interpretation, however, has varied throughout history. The term "hysteria" comes from the Greek word *hysteron,* which means the uterus or womb. Hippocrates thought that the uterus was a peregrinating organ whose wandering about the woman's body caused the malady. Sensing its relation to the sexual passions, he recommended marriage as the best remedy for it. The notion that hysteria is a condition that affects only women had thus been firmly established and was not seriously challenged until the latter half of the nineteenth century by the famed French neurologist-neuropathologist Jean-Martin Charcot.

During the first ten centuries of Christianity, medical thought stagnated under the influence of Galenic teaching. As the perspective on sickness changed from naturalistic to theological-demonological, the phenomena associated with hysteria began to be interpreted as a manifestation of witchcraft. Following the Renaissance, hysteria was "rediscovered" as a disease: in the eighteenth century, it was attributed to emotions, passions, and human suggestibility, and in the early part of the nineteenth century, to organic dysfunction. It fell to Jean-Martin Charcot, Pierre Janet, and Sigmund Freud to clarify the distinction between neurological illness and hysteria. They believed that hysteria is a condition resembling physical disease that occurs in persons with healthy bodies. If this was to be considered a genuine disease, it is easy to see why it had to be distinguished from malingering: this was accomplished by defining hysteria as the unconscious imitation of illness and malingering as the conscious imitation of it.

It is but a small step from the psychoanalytic view of hysteria, which regards it as a form of illness albeit without physical causation, to the linguistic view of it, which regards it as a form of communication, specifically, as the language of illness.

II

The claim that hysteria is an organic disease has the merit of being logical. People diagnosed as hysteric act sick and look sick, say they are ill, and are, or appear to be, disabled. In the past—the supporters of this view argue— people have been disabled by certain conditions, such as diabetes and neuro- syphilis, that were not understood as diseases until modern times. Hysteria, in this view, is another such disease: today we understand only its "mental symptoms"; research will demonstrate its physiological causation. In short, hysteria is a disease that happens to a person's body: someone suffers from it and may be cured of it. Logically, this view is sound. Factually, it is false.

Most psychiatrists who regard hysteria as an illness qualify it as a mental illness. Its pathology, therefore, is sought not in the patient's brain but in his psyche: it is a form of psychopathology. Specifically, hysterical bodily signs are believed to represent an unconscious conversion of repressed ideas, feelings, or conflicts into bodily symptoms. This explanation is also unsatisfactory.

Sigmund Freud became famous in part for his psychological theory of hysteria. Working as a physician, he developed his ideas about the "disease" to help him cope with the practical problems he faced. What were those problems? Here is Freud's own account:

> In the autumn of 1892, I was asked by a doctor I knew to examine a young lady who had been suffering for more than two years from pains in her legs and who had difficulties in walking. . . . All that was apparent was that she complained of great pain in walking and of being quickly overcome by fatigue both in walking and . . . standing, and that after a short time she had to rest . . . I did not find it easy to arrive at a diagnosis, but I decided for two reasons to assent to the one proposed by my colleague, viz. that it was a case of hysteria.[1]

What was wrong with this young woman? Freud believed that she was free of any bodily disease and concluded that she suffered from the disease called "hys- teria." How is this disease brought into being? This was Freud's explanation:

> According to the view suggested by the conversion theory what happened may be described as follows: She repressed her erotic idea from consciousness and

transformed the amount of its affect into physical sensations of pain. We may ask: What is it that turns into physical pain here? A cautious reply would be: Something that might have become, and should have become, mental pain. If we venture a little further and try to represent the ideational mechanism into a kind of algebraical picture, we may attribute a certain quota of affect to the ideational complex of these erotic feelings which remained unconscious, and say that this quantity (the quota of affect) is what was converted.[2]

Subsequently, the mechanism of the "pathogenesis of hysteria" was refined by Freud and other psychoanalysts and came to include the following "etiological factors":

• Somatic compliance. Symptoms are localized in accordance with the distribution and fixation of body libido: body parts or organs overlibidinized by previous organic disease or continuous hyperfunction become the media of expression.

• Frustration, introversion, and regression. If there is frustration of instinctual drives in adult life, the libido tends to turn from reality to fantasy. Fantasy is subject to the laws of regression.

• Reactivation of the Oedipus situation. Infantile fantasies, especially those associated with the Oedipus complex, are reactivated through regression.

• Breakdown of repression. Repression, faulty to begin with, cannot cope with the additional charge of the reactivated infantile fantasies. The defense crumbles and the repressed content breaks through: the return of the repressed.

• Symptom formation through displacement and symbolization. The specific form of conversion symptoms is determined partly by the degree of genital symbolization of various body parts, and partly by the person's unconscious identification with his incestuous objects.

The result, the psychoanalysts maintained, is an inhibition or exaggeration of bodily functions, giving rise to crippling or painful symptoms. These constitute a somatic dramatization of unconscious fantasies.

III

People often ask: Is hysteria the same today as it has always been or has its character changed during the past fifty or hundred years? Is it less common now than it was in the past? The answer depends on our concept of hysteria.

Sometimes it is claimed that hysteria was more common in Europe toward the end of the nineteenth century than it is in America today. The evidence for this view is unconvincing. What has changed is not hysteria but the sociology of medical practice. In Vienna in the 1880s, persons with bodily complaints consulted general practitioners. The doctor's job was to make a differential diagnosis between organic disease, such as neurosyphilis, and imaginary or mental disease, typically hysteria. Today, such patients still seek the help of the medical practitioner, even though, since then, a new medical specialty has arisen, namely, outpatient or office psychiatry. Because hysterical patients consider themselves medically, not mentally ill, they do not usually consult psychiatrists.

As psychiatry became a separate discipline, hysteria became a psychiatric diagnosis, presumably attached to psychiatric patients. However, persons who consult psychiatrists voluntarily or are committed to their care involuntarily rarely suffer from what appear to be bodily illnesses; more often, they feel anguished or annoy others. It is true, then, that hysteria is not particularly common among the contemporary psychiatrist's patients. This does not mean that the "incidence of hysteria" in the population at large has decreased. I believe it has not.

To be sure, persons imitating illness, communicating with others in the language of disease, do not crowd the psychoanalyst's private office. They go, instead, to shops that display the sign "Here we speak the language of illness," as Eastern European shops before the war displayed the sign, "*Ici on parle français.*" Where are such signs displayed? In the offices of general practitioners, internists, dermatologists, and neurologists; in famous diagnostic centers; in clinics where compensation for illness is awarded, such as those operated by the Veterans Administration; and in the offices of lawyers and in courts, where money damages may be sought and obtained for illness both organic and mental, real and counterfeit.

Because of such changes in the sociology of medical and psychiatric practice during the past half century, it is misleading to speak simply of the incidence of hysteria. We must specify the particular social situation in which the incidence of the alleged disorder is to be established.

IV

The psychoanalytic view of hysteria contains the germ of the communicational understanding of it, as I describe in my book *The Myth of Mental Illness*. I regard so-called hysterical symptoms as a type of communication or language, used in a context of game playing: hysterics *act* disabled and sick; their illness is not real but an *imitation* of a bodily illness. Because the hysteric impersonates the sick role, the result is "genuine" disability. If we call this condition an "illness," we use the term metaphorically, whether we realize it or not. By means of body language, hysterics communicate with themselves and others, especially those willing, perhaps even eager, to assume the role of protecting and controlling them.

Understanding the linguistic-semiotic perspective on hysteria requires a measure of familiarity with certain technical concepts, which I shall summarize. Anything in nature may or may not be a sign, depending on a person's attitude toward it. A physical thing—a chalk mark, a dark cloud, a paralyzed arm—is a sign when it appears as a substitute for the object for which it stands with respect to the sign user. The three-part relation of sign, object, and sign user is called the relation of denotation.

Linguists distinguish three classes of signs: indexical, iconic, and symbolic. In the indexical class belong signs that acquire their sign function through a causal connection. For example, smoke is a sign of fire and fever a sign of infectious disease. In the iconic class belong signs that acquire their sign function through similarity. For example, a photograph is a sign of the person in the picture; a map is a sign of the territory it represents. In the third class, symbolic, or conventional, signs, belong signs that acquire their sign function through arbitrary convention and common agreement—for example, words and mathematical symbols. Symbols do not usually exist in isolation but are coordinated with each other by a set of rules called the "rules of language." The entire package, consisting of symbols, language rules, and social customs of language use, is sometimes referred to as the "language game."

Communicational situations may comprise one, two, three, or a multitude of people. A semiotic and game-playing view of hysteria does not imply a purely social approach and therefore a neglect of the intrapersonal dimension of the phenomenon. Thus, hysteria—and other so-called mental illnesses—may occur in a one-person situation. An individual who feels abdominal pain and concludes, falsely, that it is caused by acute appendicitis illustrates this phenomenon. Such a person fools himself, not others. He plays a game by disguising his personal problem as a medical disease. The advantage derived from such a one-person game corresponds closely to the psychoanalytic idea of primary gain.

However, humans are not solitary beings. People generally do not live in isolation. Therefore the interpersonal and social aspects of "hysterical communications" are the most practically relevant. For example, if a person complains to a physician of abdominal pain and insists that it is due to an inflamed appendix even though there is no other evidence to support this view, his interpretation will first be discredited, then he himself will be discredited. The more he enlarges the social situation where he makes this false claim, the more he risks being seriously discredited by being labeled schizophrenic and committed to a mental hospital. In a manner of speaking, such a person plays a game of fooling others. To the extent that he succeeds and is accepted as sick, he profits from his strategy. This advantage corresponds closely to the psychoanalytic idea of secondary gain.

From a communicational point of view, the traditional medical problem of differentiating disease from nondisease is distinguishing iconic signs from indexical signs. The physician observes signs not diseases; the latter is an inference drawn from the former. How do we distinguish indexical signs from iconic signs? By ascertaining whether the sign is "given" by a person or "given off" by him. Iconic signs resemble conventional signs: both are manufactured, more or less deliberately, by an agent, that is a person, whereas indexical signs are given off passively by an organism or thing.

If a person complains of abdominal pain, we ought not to ask, "Is he suffering from appendicitis or hysteria?" We ought to ask, "Is the pain an indexical sign or iconic sign of an inflamed appendix? Clearly, it could be both at once. This is why it is not possible to make a "diagnosis" of hysteria by ruling out organic illness nor to make a diagnosis of organic illness by ruling out hysteria. Instead, in doubtful cases, patient and physician alike must decide whether to approach the sign as though it were indexical, signaling a disease of the body, or as though it were iconic, signaling a complaint about the self and others. The former approach requires medical investigation and treatment, the latter resembles ordinary communication.

What are the implications of taking seriously the semiotic perspective on hysteria and so-called mental illnesses generally? To begin with, we would have to personalize "hysteria" and recognize that the hysterical person is a forger, a cheat who impersonates the sick role. Next, we would have to conceive of hysteria as a dialect of the language of sickness, a form of communication especially appropriate to medical situations in which persons endeavor to define themselves as sick or disabled. The language of hysteria is composed of iconic signs, is nondiscursive, and hence easily misunderstood or misinterpreted by the receiver. This may be useful to the sender, the receiver, or both. In short, the language of hysteria is a type of rhetoric, useful for inducing strong feeling in others and an urge to action; it is not a type of dialectic, useful for conveying accurate information.

What do I mean when I assert that hysteria is a form of rhetoric? Let us examine what he, or she, *does*. He complains of pain and suffering, exhibits bodily signs suggesting that he is sick, and arouses and alarms those about him. He does all this by confronting them with what seems like a desperate situation requiring immediate intervention. Why does he do this? Because he knows that he lacks a legitimate ground for making demands on others and knows that the language of illness is more effective as a rhetorical device than the language of everyday speech.

To identify a person, we use his photograph or fingerprint, not a verbal description of his appearance. The hysteric uses a similar principle. If one person seeks the attention or help of another individual, he can achieve his aim best by a dramatic display of messages that say, in effect, "I am sick! I am helpless! You must help me!" This goal is better accomplished by displaying the image or icon of illness—a seemingly sick body—than by simply stating that one feels ill. A picture is worth a thousand words. A hysterical symptom is worth two thousand. That sums up the rhetoric of hysteria.

V

The implications of a linguistic theory of hysteria are most far-reaching for its so-called treatment, a term whose literal meaning applies only to somatic medicine. A disease may be cured. A person may be coerced or influenced to conform or change himself.

Does the hysteric want to be changed? Often he does not. He prefers to change others. This insight, poorly understood and even more poorly articulated, led many physicians in the past to conclude that such patients were "social parasites" who, in the words of an early-twentieth-century French writer, "would . . . steal anything conveniently within reach, lie, cheat, make work and trouble for others."[3]

Because hysteria is a form of rhetoric, it often evokes a counterrhetorical response. The patient tries to coerce through symptoms. The physician tries to coerce through hypnosis. The result is often a mutually antagonistic, mutually deceptive relationship. Sometimes the patient dominates, sometimes the doctor does, and sometimes the contest ends in a draw. Psychoanalysis sought to transcend this interpersonal impasse by substituting dialectic for rhetoric, discursive language for nondiscursive.

It may also happen that the physician, wittingly or unwittingly, treats the hysteric as if he, or she, were truly ill. The physician accepts the patient's communications couched in the language of illness and replies in the same idiom. In the past, this took the form of mythical diagnoses, such as retroflexion of the uterus or focal infection. The value of the treatment, often surgical, lay in legitimating the patient's occupancy of the sick role, not in ameliorating a disease. Today, it is easier than ever to treat the hysterical person as if he or she were ill: that is what the new psychotropic drugs are for.

10

Routine Neonatal Circumcision

A Medical Ritual

I realized that ritual will always mean throwing away something;
Destroying our corn or wine upon the altar of our gods.
—Gilbert K. Chesterton,
Tremendous Trifles (1909)

I

THERE IS A VAST LITERATURE on the medical arguments for and
against the practice of routine neonatal circumcision (RNC). My aim here
is not to join that debate but rather to identify the ethical dilemma that a
dispassionate examination of RNC forces upon us. I shall show that RNC
appears to be a medical-prophylactic procedure because, in the United States
today, it is usually performed by physicians. In fact, it is a Jewish and Muslim
religious ritual.

Formerly, religious rituals and rationalizations imparted meaning to
people's lives and justified controlling their conduct. Today, medical rituals
and rationalization perform those functions. When suicide, for example,
was viewed as self-murder, the actor's sinning justified imposing priestly
sanctions on his corpse. When the desire for suicide is viewed as a manifestation of mental illness, the actor's disease justifies imposing psychiatric
sanctions on his person. Homosexuality and masturbation are two other
common behaviors that were first forbidden on religious grounds and then
on medical grounds.

While homosexuality, masturbation, and suicide are behaviors, being
born a male is not. Accordingly, circumcision is justified not by the subject's

behavior but by the significance his parents and society attach to his foreskin. For Jews, the ritual sacrifice of the infant's foreskin symbolizes his entrance into the community of the chosen. For educated Americans, its prophylactic removal symbolizes his entrance into the community of the medically enlightened. Indeed, *Webster's* defines circumcision as "The cutting off of the prepuce of males being practiced as a religious rite by Jews and Muslims *and* as a sanitary measure in modern surgery" (emphasis added).

II

The biblical origin of circumcision is the covenant between God and Abraham: "And God said to Abraham, . . . 'This is my covenant, which you shall keep, between me and you and your descendants after you: Every male among you shall be circumcised. . . . Any uncircumcised male who is not circumcised in the flesh of his foreskin shall be cut off from his people; he has broken my covenant.'"[1] The ancient Israelites made a bargain with their god: they gave Jehovah their foreskins in return for which Jehovah gave them preferred nation status. It seems likely that the ritual circumcision of the male infant is an attenuated version of child sacrifice.

The idea that there is a hygienic basis for this biblical rule is inconsistent with the passage depicting the enemy's severed penile foreskin as a trophy:

> Then Saul said, "Thus shall you say to David, 'The king desires no marriage present except a hundred foreskins of the Philistines, that he may be avenged of the king's enemies.'" . . . Before the time had expired, David arose and went, along with his men, and killed two hundred of the Philistines; and David brought their foreskins, which were given in full number to the king, that he might become the king's son-in-law.[2]

The magical powers attributed to manipulating the penile foreskin are further illustrated by the following Talmudic story: "In the Hereafter Abraham will sit at the entrance of *Gehinnom* [Hell] and will not allow any circumcised Israelite to descend into it. As for those who sinned unduly, what does he do to them? He removes the foreskin from children who had died before circumcision, places it upon them and send them down to *Gehinnom*."[3]

To justify expelling the deviant from the group, he must first be transformed into the Other: before consigning the sinful Jew to hell, he is restored to his uncircumcised state; before committing the sick patient to the mental hospital, he is declared "dangerous to himself or others."[4] Every social group distinguishes between persons who are members of the group and those who are not. Jews base that distinction on circumcision, symbolizing their covenant with God. This is why Orthodox Jews circumcise dead infants: the ritual insures that, when they are resurrected, they will be members of the chosen people. We base it on mental health, symbolizing the individual's capacity to covenant (contract) with other members of society. (I ignore citizenship here as a marker of membership in the in-group.)

That the practice of circumcision has its origin in ritual is so incontrovertible that not even the most zealous advocates of the procedure try to deny it. They do, however, try to rationalize it—much as people have tried to rationalize the Jewish dietary laws—as an expression of primitive insight into its hygienic character. However, ritual circumcision flies in the face of the most elementary principles of hygiene. Traditional Jewish law requires the circumciser, called "mohel," to perform the ritual act of *metzitzah,* which consists of his taking the circumcised penis in his mouth and sucking out the blood, an act that must be repeated three times. Around the turn of the century, concerns over the documented spread of tuberculosis and syphilis from mohel to infant caused American Jews largely to abandon this element of the ritual. As recently as 1962, Charles Weiss, writing in *Clinical Pediatrics,* felt it necessary to repeat the call to outlaw this practice.[5] In France, legislation enacted in 1845 prohibited the practice of *metzitzah* and mandated that circumcision "be performed in a rational manner."[6]

The Torah, Talmud, and the body of historical Jewish thought all are very clear about the origins and nature of circumcision. The great Jewish philosopher and rabbi Moses Maimonides (1135–1204) stated the case clearly: "No one, however, should circumcise himself or his son for any other reason but pure faith."[7] Modern efforts to attribute medical rationale to this primitive practice have no basis in scholarship and are disrespectful of Jewish tradition.

III

How and when did ritual circumcision become prophylactic circumcision, and why did it become especially popular in the United States? For millennia, neither circumcision nor the delivery of the pregnant woman was considered to be a medical procedure. The penile foreskin was regarded as a normal body part, and pregnancy was regarded as a normal event. Women gave birth unassisted or were delivered by female relatives or by informally trained midwives. So long as that remained the practice, circumcision could not become a medical procedure. Much has been written about the conquest of pregnancy and delivery for medicine, male professionals displacing female amateurs as the sole legally authorized providers of so-called obstetrical services.[8] Along with this change, the place of delivery was transferred from the home to the hospital, and normal birth itself came to be seen as a surgical intervention, supposedly facilitated by routine episiotomy. The stage was set for the routine surgical circumcision of the normal male infant by the obstetrician, rationalized as prophylaxis. Against what? The answer is masturbation, a plague that could be prevented as well as cured by circumcision.

Virtually all medical texts at the end of the nineteenth century and the beginning of the twentieth prescribed circumcision for a variety of ills, ranging from epilepsy and hydrocephalus to malnutrition and tuberculosis, and confidently asserted that it was a cure for the "disease" of masturbation. The following statement from a standard medical text published in 1887 is typical: "Whether masturbation is a cause of epilepsy is doubted. But there can be no doubt of its injurious effect. . . . *Circumcision should always be practiced.* It may be necessary to make the genital so sore by blistering fluids that pain results from attempts to rub the part."[9]

Many critics of RNC recognize that beliefs about masturbation played a part in the advent of this practice. They fail to appreciate, however, that the American enthusiasm for preventing masturbation and for promoting circumcision are manifestations of the same puritanical zeal for health as virtue that has fueled other typically American crowd madnesses, such as Prohibition, the war on drugs, and the mental health movement.[10] For example, Edward Wallerstein, the author of *Circumcision: An American Health Fallacy*,[11] writes, "So-called 'health' circumcision originated in the nineteenth century. . . . Within the miasma of myth and ignorance, a theory emerged that masturbation caused many and varied ills."[12] This statement barely hints at the role of the myth of masturbatory insanity, a genuine crowd madness that began in the eighteenth century, long before RNC appeared, quickly became irresistible medical dogma in both Europe and the United States, and disappeared only in the middle of the twentieth century. Since then, medical hysteria has shifted from masturbation to other health hazards, such as smoking and obesity. Today, circumcision is considered as a "strategy for AIDS prevention."[13]

The significance of the idea of masturbatory insanity lies in the fact that sexual self-stimulation was the first in a long line of religious transgressions converted into medical diseases. The roots of both RNC and antimasturbatory measures lie in Jewish law, which recognizes the legitimacy of erotic pleasure associated with sexual intercourse provided that the act is marital-genital congress between a Jewish man and a Jewish woman. Every other sexual act is strictly prohibited. Masturbation is condemned unequivocally both in the Talmud and in extra-Talmudic literature. The *Zohar* (an authoritative commentary on the Pentateuch) calls masturbation "a sin more serious than all the sins of the Torah."[14] Jewish exegetes interpret the act as murder and say that the guilty person deserves death, a hyperbole indicating that the prohibition rests on the view that, by destroying his "generative seed," the masturbator commits an act not unlike murder. Recognizing the obvious connections between touching the penis and sexual arousal, Jewish law "definitely prohibits touching one's genitals—the unmarried man never, and the married man only in connection with urination."[15] When an orthodox Jewish father bladder trains his son, he admonishes him, "Without hands! Better a bad aim than a bad habit." For a male to urinate without hands is a difficult enough feat if he is circumcised. If he is not, it is virtually impossible. The relevance for RNC of the connection between the prohibition against possessing penile foreskin and against touching the penis while urinating has not received the attention it deserves. This, then, is the background against which we must view the history of the antimasturbation movement and its corollary, medical circumcision.

The credit for inventing and successfully popularizing the idea that masturbation poses a grave hazard to health belongs to an anonymous clergyman-physician who, in 1710, published a treatise entitled *Onania, or the Heinous Sin of Self-Pollution*.[16] This was followed, in 1758, by the publication of *Onania, Or a Treatise upon the Disorders Produced by Masturbation*, by Simon-André Tissot, a prominent physician in Lausanne. This work established masturbation as a major etiological factor in countless diseases and transformed the pathogenicity of masturbation from theory into dogma. Benjamin Rush, Philippe Pinel, Henry Maudsley, Sigmund Freud are just a few of the celebrated medical personages who never questioned the harmfulness of self-abuse.

It requires education to see the world through disease-colored glasses. Thus members of the upper classes are the most ardent consumers of medical fables, while members of the lower classes tend to be skeptical of health information, both valid and invalid.[17] The role of medical misinformation is humorously mocked in *Knock* (1923), a masterpiece by Jules Romains that is all but forgotten today. Dr. Knock explains his views as follows: "'Get sick' is an old idea. It can't stand up to modern science. 'Health' is a word which we could just as well erase from our vocabularies. For me there are only people more or less sick of more or less numerous diseases progressing at a more or less rapid rate. . . . A profoundly modern theory, M. Mousquet. If you think it over, you'll be struck by its relation to the admirable concept of the nation in arms, a concept from which our modern states derive their strength."[18]

This parody has become our social reality. We conceptualize every problem in living—from the misbehavior of children to the melancholia of adults—as a disease. Given this mind-set, it is not surprising that circumcision became medicalized and that RNC proved to be especially popular in the United States. It is worth noting here that in the 1950s the British National Health Service stopped paying for RNC, while American third-party payers, including welfare programs, began to reimburse the procedure and "circumcision became the American standard."[19] By 1993, the rate of circumcision dropped to 5 to 6 percent in Britain, and stood at 80 to 90 percent in the United States. Despite this, the incidence of the cancer of the penis is higher in the United States than in Denmark and Japan, "where circumcision is done only for clear medical indications."[20] This observation is valid only for the *overall* incidence of cancer of the penis in these countries.

In the United States, the incidence of cancer of the penis is much higher in men who are not circumcised than in those who are.

IV

Why is RNC legal? Because it is defined as preventive medicine. Why is it defined as preventive medicine? To avoid having to ban it as male genital mutilation. This reciprocal relationship between language and law is intrinsic to our concept of legality. Whether a particular act is legal or illegal depends on what we call it. Killing called "self-defense" is legal; killing called "murder" is a crime. We call the removal of the foreskin of the male newborn "routine neonatal circumcision" and the removal of parts of the female genitalia "female genital mutilation" (FGM). Language thus prejudges the legitimacy (or illegitimacy) of the practice.

Although neither female circumcision, or clitoridectomy, performed ostensibly to stop masturbation, nor other forms of FGM performed for cultural-religious reasons mainly in Muslim African countries is within the scope this essay, I wish to add a few brief remarks about them here. Clitoridectomy was sometimes practiced in English-speaking countries until well past World War II and, in the United States, Blue Cross–Blue Shield paid for it until 1977.[21] Female genital mutilations of all types are now banned in most European countries as well as in the United Kingdom. In the United States, the federal government and sixteen states have criminalized the practice. Although most Americans refuse to compare the two procedures, the similarities are obvious and apparent to Europeans: both interventions alter the normal anatomy of the genital organs, and the people who practice them attribute health benefits to both (Americans to male circumcision, Africans to female circumcision).[22] In Nigeria, 21.2 percent of female circumcisions are performed by physicians.[23]

In 1949, an editorial in the *British Medical Journal* condemned RNC as an intervention that "savours of the barbaric," reemphasized its essentially religious-ritual character by listing some of the "bizarre" methods that people have used for disposing of the amputated foreskin, and strongly criticized physicians for permitting the practice.[24] In 1976, in an important paper in *Pediatrics,* William F. Gee and Julian S. Ansell refuted the cancer-protective powers sometimes attributed to the procedure: "Circumcision has been justified on the basis that carcinoma of the penis is rare in circumcised males. However, if one compares the incidence of carcinoma of the penis in comparable circumcised and uncircumcised white, male populations in temperate zones in Scandinavia versus the United States, there is no significant difference in the incidence of carcinoma of the penis (1/100,000) between those circumcised and those not circumcised."[25]

In 1989, the Task Force on Circumcision of the American Academy of Pediatrics (a group reserved about the benefits of RNC) nevertheless still cited the lower incidence of cancer of the penis in circumcised males as justifying the practice.[26] Although it recognized that poor genital hygiene plays a role in the etiology of this disease, the task force failed to mention that even if circumcision offers protection from penile cancer, it cannot justify its routine use before the age of consent. Cancer of the penis is a rare condition that occurs only in middle age or later, affording young males who fear developing the disease time to submit to prophylactic circumcision. Other pathological conditions associated with the uncircumcised penis, such as phimosis severe enough to interfere with urination and urinary tract infections, are indications for treating the affected children, not for RNC.

In short, the medical rationalization of mass circumcision is one of the most obvious and most overlooked illustrations of our acculturation to the ideology of the therapeutic state. No longer advocated for the prevention of masturbation, circumcision is now regarded as the standard prophylactic measure against penile cancer and urinary tract infections. Although the cause of penile cancer is unknown, it seems unlikely that it lies in the normal anatomy of the human male. Moreover, the claim that later circumcision offers less protection against penile cancer than neonatal circumcision, typically advanced by supporters of RNC, rests on the misleading comparison of penile cancer rates in Jews and Moslems. Jews circumcise on the eighth day of life; Moslems, at puberty. It is known that hygiene and venereal disease play a role in the causation of penile cancer; and that, for a variety of cultural and economic reasons, Jews generally have higher hygienic standards and lower rates of venereal disease than Moslems. Therefore, despite claims to the contrary, the idea that only RNC offers protection against cancer of the penis remains unproven.[27]

The claim that RNC is rational prophylaxis against urinary tract infections (UTI) is also inconsistent with the evidence. According to a recent study, 99.8 percent of circumcised infants, and 98.6 percent of uncircumcised infants never experience this (easily diagnosed and treated) problem.[28] Thus, the most that RNC can be credited for is that it reduces the rate of UTI in infants by 1.2 percent.

The conclusion of two Swedish physicians seems to me sound: "With regard to prevention of diseases in adult men, it is in our opinion more fair to postpone a decision [about circumcision] till the young male can make a choice of his own."[29]

V

I believe the time has come to acknowledge that the practice of RNC rests on the absurd premise that the only mammal in creation born in a condition that requires immediate surgical correction is the human male. If the penile foreskin is not merely nonfunctional but a biological disadvantage so severe as to justify its immediate surgical ablation, then, surely, it might have atrophied by now. Accordingly, it is not enough for physicians to conclude—as the author of a comment in 1990, in the *New England Journal of Medicine,* concludes, "[T]he benefits [of circumcision] appear to be uncertain. It, therefore, seems prudent to consider neonatal circumcision a procedure to be performed at the discretion of parents, not as a part of routine medical care. Omitting circumcision in the neonatal period should not be considered medical neglect. Parents should be informed of the current state of medical knowledge regarding the risks and benefits of the procedure. *Their ultimate decision may hinge on nonmedical considerations.*"[30]

If the parents' ultimate decision to circumcise their male infant hinges on nonmedical considerations, then RNC is a medically unjustifiable practice. It is relevant to note in this connection that observant Jewish parents still employ mohels to circumcise their male infants, a practice the American Medical Association (AMA) explicitly endorses. The AMA's Law Department provides a special "Release for Ritual Circumcision" form for "parents of Jewish faith [who] request the performance of a circumcision by a person other than a physician." Executed by the infant's parents, the document

authorizes the attending physician and hospital "to permit our son to be circumcised by —— whom we have selected as a person qualified in the ritual
of our faith and by experience to perform this procedure."[31] What entitles
the parents of a Jewish male infant to authorize a nonphysician—who is a
religious personage to boot—to perform a surgical procedure? Practicing
medicine without a license is a criminal offense. Accordingly, circumcision
by a mohel is a crime, and since he is a religious official, it is also a violation
of the separation of church and state.

If RNC is medically unjustifiable, does it constitute a form of child
abuse? Persons unbound by Jewish and Islamic religious rules might reach
that conclusion.[32] Should it be illegal? Therein lies our ethical dilemma. We
must balance the (relatively small) harm RNC does to the individual against
the (potentially vast) harm that strengthening the state at the expense of the
family does to everyone. Because the family remains our most secure shield
against the encroachments of the therapeutic state, the dilemma calls for
compromise. Preventing RNC does not warrant enlisting the coercive apparatus of state against the religious values of parents. It does warrant, however, enlisting the persuasive powers of physicians in the task of informing
parents of newborn males about the medically dubious and morally problematic nature of this ostensibly hygienic procedure.

11

The Fatal Temptation

Drug Control and Suicide

[T]he government offers to cure all the ills of mankind. . . . All that is
needed is to create some new government agencies and to pay a few more
bureaucrats. In a word, the tactic consists in initiating, in the guise of
actual services, what are nothing but restrictions; thereafter, the nation
pays, not for being served, but for being disserved.

—Frédéric Bastiat, *Economic Sophisms* (1845)

I

IN AMERICA, quipped Will Rogers, "Everything has a slogan, and of all
the bunk in America, the slogan is the champ . . . Congress even has slogans:
'Why sleep at home, when you can sleep in Congress?' 'Be a politician—no
training necessary!'"[1]

I would add that of all the bunk in America, our champion slogans
are about drugs and medical ethics: "Just say no to drugs," "the sanctity
of life," "pro-choice," "the right to life," "the right to die," "the right to
treatment," "the right to reject treatment"—slogans all, some contradicting
others and yet all coexisting comfortably in mindless harmony. If the right
to autonomy—to our bodies, minds, and selves—means anything, it means a
right to suicide. And if pro-choice means anything, it must mean the right to
use or abstain from using any particular drug. And yet these are precisely the
rights no normal American endorses. Indeed, we are so phobic about suicide
that we fear even knowing about it. According to a survey reported in the
May 18, 1992, issue of *U.S. News and World Report,* 71 percent of Americans would like libraries to ban "books describing how to commit suicide."[2]

I suggest, then, that fear of the temptation to commit suicide is a critical, yet rarely considered, facet of drug controls.

The right to do X does not means that doing X is morally meritorious. We have a right to divorce our spouse, vote for a politician we know nothing about, eat until we are obese, or squander our money on lottery tickets. Thus, the phrase "right to suicide" does not mean that suicide is a morally desirable or meritorious act. It means only that agents of the state have no right or power to interfere, by prohibitions or punishments, with a person's decision to kill himself. Those who desire to prevent a particular person from committing suicide must content themselves with their power, such as it might be, to persuade him to change his mind.

II

Because we have a free market in food, we can buy all the bacon, eggs, and ice cream we want and can afford. If we had a free market in drugs, we could similarly buy all the barbiturates, chloral hydrate, and morphine we want and could afford. We would then be free to die, easily, comfortably, and surely—without any need for recourse to death doctors or violent means of suicide, and without fear of being kept alive against our will to die a protracted, painful, and extravagantly expensive death in a building misnamed a "hospital." We would then no longer have to complain about doctors, nurses, relatives, hospitals, and courts overtreating us, undertreating us, withholding pain medications from us, keeping us alive, and depriving us of our "right to die."[3]

How did the idea of a "right to die" arise? How can the inevitable biological destiny of all living beings be a right? What does the phrase mean? Actually, the phrase refers primarily to our confused rejection of the spectacle of doctors keeping moribund persons alive with the aid of modern biotechnological machinery. Why do physicians do this? Because they enjoy the powers science and the state have put in their hands, because they often have both professional and economic incentives for it, because they assume that is what the patient would want, because courts or kin command them to do "everything possible" to keep the patient alive, and, lastly, because withholding life-sustaining measures could be regarded as deliberately killing the patient. In short, we prattle about a "right to die" because we prefer mouthing uplifting slogans to thinking seriously about the meaning of life.

For most of us today, the term "sanctity of life" has lost virtually all meaning. We cling to life—up to a point. After that, we want to be "allowed" to die—an imagery that falsely implies that we are inescapably bound to persons determined to prevent us from dying. To deny them that role, we have complemented the proposition that we have a "right to life" (which has become the code phrase of the antiabortion movement), with the seemingly contrary proposition that we have a "right to die."

However, the similarity between these two semantically reciprocal rights is illusory. Each addresses a completely different set of existential choices and ethical perplexities. The phrase "right to life" refers to the ("natural") inception of life; moreover, this "right" is ascribed to *all* unborn fetuses and belongs to each unconditionally. In contrast, the phrase "right to die" refers to the ("unnatural") termination of life, and this "right" is ascribed *only* to terminally ill persons and, in practice, often belongs to their relatives.

Thus, the phrase "right to die" is emblematic not only of our skittishness about suicide and our longing for good doctors to kill us at just the right time and in just the right way but, more fundamentally, of our repudiation of bodily self-ownership and the responsibilities that go with it. It remains to be seen how many Americans prefer legalizing doctors to kill them to legalizing themselves to own drugs, and shouldering the responsibilities that the ownership of such a valuable property entails.

So long as the phrase "right to die" does not include an unqualified right to suicide—a subject its supporters never mention—it is destined to be nothing more or less than just another step in the medicalization of life and in our headlong rush into the deadly embrace of the therapeutic state. On the other hand, if the phrase is intended to encompass the right to suicide, then—lest it be an empty slogan—the "right to die" must include the "right to drugs." We know, however, that most people—especially in the United States—consider the desire to commit suicide, much less the act itself, not a right but a symptom of preventable and treatable mental illness. As against this view, I hold that the option to commit suicide is inherent in the human condition, that committing suicide ought to be considered a basic human right and may sometimes be a moral duty, and the expectation or threat of suicide never justifies the coercive control of the (allegedly) suicidal person. At the same time, I consider it a basic moral wrong for a physician to kill a patient, or anyone else, and call it "euthanasia."[4] This does not mean that "pulling the plug" on a dying patient is (necessarily) an immoral act; it means only that doing so does not (necessarily) require medical expertise, should not be defined as a medical intervention, and should not be delegated (specifically) to physicians. I maintain that our longing for doctors to give us lethal drugs betokens our desire to evade responsibility for giving such drugs to ourselves. So long as we are more interested in investing doctors with the right to kill than in reclaiming our own right to drugs, our discourse about rights and drugs is destined to remain empty, meaningless chatter.

Of course, a people cannot expect to regain their right to acts and objects unless they are willing and prepared to assume responsibility for the conduct of the acts and the care of the objects in question. Since the most important practical consequence of our loss of the right to bodily self-ownership is the denial of legally unrestricted access to drugs, the most important symbol of the right to our bodies now resides in our reasserting our right to drugs—to all drugs, not just to one or another so-called recreational drug. At this point, we come face-to-face with our real drug problem—namely, that most Americans today do not want to have legally unrestricted access to drugs. On the contrary, they dread the idea and the prospect it portends.

In sum, we have launched ourselves on a self-contradictory quest, for an America where no one "abuses" drugs because doctors effectively control drug use and where everyone dies a painless and pleasant death because doctors compassionately kill "dying" people who want to be killed. Having combined a dread of dying a protracted, pointless, and perhaps painful death with a fear of living with a free market in drugs, we have negated our chances for attaining pharmacological autonomy, that is, freedom and responsibility vis-à-vis the drugs we take similar to the freedom and responsibility we have vis-à-vis the foods we eat, the books we read, and the religion we profess.

12

Pedophilia Therapy

History consists for the greater part of the miseries brought upon the world by pride, ambition, avarice, revenge, lust, sedition, hypocrisy, ungoverned zeal, and all the train of disorderly appetites which shake the public.... These vices are the *causes* of those storms. Religion, morals, laws, prerogatives, privileges, liberties, rights of men are the *pretexts*. The pretexts are always found in some specious appearance of a real good.... As these are the pretexts, so the ordinary actors and instruments in great public evils are kings, priests, magistrates, senates, parliaments, national assemblies, judges, and captains.... A certain quantum of power must always exist in the community in some hands and under some appellation. Wise men will apply their remedies to vices, not to names; to the causes of evil which are permanent, not to the occasional organs by which they act, and the transitory modes in which they appear.

—Edmund Burke, *Reflections*
on the Revolution in France (1790)

I

WE USE WORDS to label and help us comprehend the world around us. However, many of the words we use are like distorting lenses: they make us misperceive and hence misjudge the object we look at. As Sir James Fitzjames Stephen, the great nineteenth-century English jurist, aptly put it, "Men have an all but incurable propensity to prejudge all the great questions which interest them by stamping their prejudices upon their language." This is especially true when we label a sexual behavior a disease, because the word "disease" combines a description with a (covert) value judgment.

Consider the ongoing scandal involving Roman Catholic priests accused of molesting boys. American law defines sexual congress between an adult and a child as a crime. The American Psychiatric Association defines it as a disease and calls it "pedophilia."

Crimes are acts we commit. Diseases are biological processes that happen to our bodies. Mixing these two concepts—and defining behaviors we disapprove of as diseases—is a bottomless source of confusion and corruption.

That confusion was illustrated by a February 8 letter to the *Boston Globe*, in which the Rev. John F. Burns defended Boston cardinal Bernard Law against critics who said he ought to resign. As an archbishop, Law had transferred the Rev. John J. Geoghan to a new parish despite allegations of sexual abuse. Geoghan eventually was accused of molesting more than 100 children over three decades. "It should be noted that neither Cardinal Bernard Law nor Father John Geoghan was aware early on of the etiology or pathology of the disease of pedophilia," Burns wrote. "The cardinal did what an archbishop does best. He showed kindness and love to an apparent errant priest. Father Geoghan also did what more recent knowledge shows pedophiles do: namely, be in total denial, with hardly any remembrance or remorse for their diseased acts. Calling for the cardinal's resignation is absurd. Let the healing begin and the law take its course."

The law is taking its course, and not only in the suits filed against the church by the victims of Geoghan and other abusive priests. Geoghan himself has been convicted of molestation in one case and faces trial in another. But if his behavior was caused by "the disease of pedophilia," a condition that not only compelled him to fondle boys but erased his memory of those "diseased acts," how can it be just to punish him? The uncertainty introduced by viewing sexual abuse as the symptom of a disease played an important role in the church's failure to protect congregants from priests like Geoghan. In a May 8 deposition, Cardinal Law was asked how he approached molestation charges. "I viewed this as a pathology, as a psychological pathology, as an illness," he said. "Obviously, I viewed it as something that had a moral component. It was, objectively speaking, a gravely sinful act." The combination of these two irreconcilable views, medical and moral, was a recipe for inaction.

II

Today virtually any unwanted behavior, from shopaholism and kleptomania to sexaholism and pedophilia, may be defined as a disease whose diagnosis and treatment belong in the province of the medical system. Disease-making thus has become similar to lawmaking. Politicians, responsive to tradition and popular opinion, can define any act, from teaching slaves to read to the cold-blooded murder of a bank guard, as a crime whose control belongs in the province of the criminal justice system.

Applied to behavior, especially sexual behavior, the disease label combines a description with a covert value judgment. Masturbation, homosexuality, and the use of nongenital body parts (especially the mouth and anus) for sexual gratification have, at one time or place, all been considered sins, crimes, diseases, normal behaviors, and even therapeutic measures. For many years psychiatrists imprisoned homosexuals and tried to "cure" them; now they self-righteously proclaim that homosexuality is normal and diagnose people who oppose that view as "homophobic." Psychiatrists diagnose the person who eats too much as suffering from "bulimia" and the person who eats too little as suffering from "anorexia nervosa." Similarly, the person who has too much sex suffers from "sex addiction," while the person who shows too little interest in sex suffers from "sexual aversion disorder." Yet psychiatrists do not consider celibacy a form of mental illness; celibate persons are not said to suffer from "anerotica nervosa."

Why not? Because psychiatrists, politicians, and the media respect the Roman Catholic Church's definition of celibacy as a virtue, a "gift from God," even though celibacy is at least as "abnormal" as homosexuality, which the church continues to define as a grievous sin—an "intrinsic evil," in the words of Cardinal Anthony Bevilacqua. Regardless of how unnatural or socially destructive a pattern of sexual behavior might be, if the church declares it to be virtuous—as with celibacy or abstinence from nonprocreative sexual acts—psychiatrists do not classify it as a disease. Thus a religion's moral teachings shape what is ostensibly a scientific judgment.

Conversely, psychiatric diagnoses affect moral judgments. Fred Berlin, the founder of the Johns Hopkins Sexual Disorders Clinic and a professor of psychiatry at the Johns Hopkins School of Medicine, declares: "Some research suggests that some genetic and hormonal abnormalities may play a role [in pedophilia]. . . . We now recognize that it's not just a moral issue, and that nobody chooses to be sexually attracted to young people." Yet an action that affects other people is always, by definition, a moral issue, regardless of whether the actor chooses the proclivity to engage in it.

Berlin misleadingly talks about the involuntariness of being "sexually attracted to young people." The issue is not sexual attraction; it is sexual action. A healthy twenty-year-old male with heterosexual interests is likely to be powerfully attracted to every halfway pretty woman he sees. This does not mean that he has, or attempts to have, sexual congress with these women, especially against their will. The entire psychiatric literature on what used to be called "sexual perversions" is permeated by the unfounded idea—always implied, sometimes asserted—that "abnormal" sexual impulses are harder to resist than "normal" ones.

The acceptance of this notion helps explain the widespread belief that sex offenders are more likely than other criminals to commit new crimes, an assumption that is not supported by the evidence. Tracking a sample of state prisoners who were released in 1983, the Bureau of Justice Statistics found that 52 percent of rapists and 48 percent of other sex offenders were arrested for a new crime within three years, compared to 60 percent of all violent offenders. The recidivism rates for nonviolent crimes were even higher: 70 percent for burglary and 78 percent for car theft, for example.

These numbers suggest that pedophiles resist their impulses more often than car thieves do. In any case, it is impossible to verify empirically whether an impulse is resistible. We can only say whether it was in fact resisted. But that doesn't matter, because the purpose of such a pseudomedical claim is to excuse the actor of moral and legal responsibility.

Catholic officials took advantage of this psychiatric absolution to avoid dealing decisively with priests who were guilty of sexual abuse. What do church authorities do when a priest is accused of molesting children? They send him to a prestigious psychiatric hospital—Johns Hopkins in Baltimore, the Institute of Living in Hartford, the Menninger Foundation in Topeka—for "treatment." In practice, the psychiatric hospital is a safe house for the sexually misbehaving priest, a place where he can be hidden until he is quietly reassigned to continue his abuse elsewhere. Berlin claims such priests are closely watched after being discharged. But a priest who commits sexual abuse is a criminal who should be imprisoned, not a patient who should be monitored by psychiatrists in the church's pay.

III

Sex with minors was not always considered a disease. In ancient Greece, sexual relationships between men and boys were a normal part of life. Such relations, called "pederastic," typically occurred between a twenty- to thirty-year-old man and a twelve- to seventeen-year-old boy. The man pursued the boy, and the boy submitted to him as the passive partner in anal sex. The man also played the role of mentor to his pupil. With the arrival of heavy pubic hair, usually at age eighteen, the younger man found a boy to mentor and get sexual satisfaction from. Sexual relations between men and young children played no part in Greek pederasty. Judaism and Christianity redefined same-sex relations as unnatural and condemned them as sinful. Then, as criminal laws supplemented or replaced ecclesiastical laws, same-sex relations became crimes as well. That understanding governed popular opinion until the rise of secularism and medical science.

The first person to propose redefining "pederasty," which in the eighteenth century became the term for what we call homosexuality, appears to have been the French physician Ambroise Tardieu (1818–1879). In 1857 Tardieu published a forensic-medical study to assist courts in cases involving pederasty. Tardieu believed that the penises of active homosexuals were anatomically different from the penises of passive homosexuals and normal people, that the anuses of passive homosexuals were anatomically different from the anuses of active homosexuals and normals, and that physicians could examine individuals and diagnose homosexuality by observing these alleged markers.

It remained for Karl Friedrich Otto Westphal (1833–1890), a famous German neurologist, to convert homosexuality from a disease identifiable by examining the subject's body into a mental illness identifiable by examining the subject's mind. Westphal renamed pederasty "sexual inversion" (in German, "contrary sexual feeling"), a term that was widely used well into the twentieth century. It was also Westphal who popularized the erroneous idea, still held by many people, that male homosexuals are effeminate and female homosexuals are masculine. He argued that since sexual inversion was a disease it should be treated by doctors rather than punished by law.

IV

Creating diseases by coining pseudomedical terms was raised to the level of an art form by Baron Richard von Krafft-Ebing (1840–1902), a German-born professor of psychiatry at the Universities of Strasbourg, Graz, and Vienna. In his *Psychopathia Sexualis* (1886), which made him world famous, Krafft-Ebing authoritatively renamed sexual sins and crimes "sexual perversions" and declared them to be "Cerebral Neuroses." Lawyers, politicians, and the public embraced this transformation as the progress of science instead of dismissing it as medical megalomania based on nothing more than the manipulation of language. "Sexology" became an integral part of medicine and the new science of psychiatry.

We have come a long way from Krafft-Ebing. In July 1998, Temple University psychologist Bruce Rind and two colleagues published their research on pedophilia in the *Psychological Bulletin,* a journal of the American Psychological Association. The authors concluded that the deleterious effects on a child of sexual relations with an adult "were neither pervasive nor typically intense." They recommended that a child's "willing encounter with positive reactions" be called "adult-child sex" instead of "abuse."

Not surprisingly, this conclusion created a furor, which led to a retraction and apology. Raymond Fowler, chief executive officer of the American Psychological Association, acknowledged that the journal's editors should have evaluated "the article based on its potential for misinforming the public policy process, but failed to do so."

Apparently no one noticed that, according to the fourth edition of the American Psychiatric Association's *Diagnostic and Statistical Manual of Mental Disorders* (*DSM-IV*, published in 1994), a person meets the criteria for pedophilia only if his "fantasies, sexual urges, or behaviors cause clinically significant distress or impairment in social, occupational, or other important areas of functioning." In short, pedophilia is a mental illness only if the actor is distressed by his actions. Psychiatrists had likewise classified homosexuality as a disease if the individual was dissatisfied with his sexual orientation ("ego-dystonic homosexuality") but not if he was satisfied with it ("ego-syntonic homosexuality"). Bending to the wind, the American Psychiatric Association later backtracked. In *DSM-IV-TR,* published in 2000, the requirement of "clinically significant distress or impairment" was omitted from the criteria for pedophilia.

Mental health professionals are not the only "progressives" eager to legitimize adult-child sex by portraying opposition to it as old-fashioned antisexual prejudice. In a 1999 article, Harris Mirkin, a professor of political science at the University of Missouri–Kansas City, stated that "children are the last bastion of the old sexual morality." As summarized by the *New York Times,* he argued that "the notion of the innocent child was a social construct, that all intergenerational sex should not be lumped into one ugly pile and that the panic over pedophilia fit a pattern of public response to female sexuality and homosexuality, both of which were once considered deviant." Mirkin cited precedents such as Greek pederasty. "Though Americans consider intergenerational sex to be evil," he wrote, "it has been permissible or obligatory in many cultures and periods of history." He told the *Times,* "I don't think it's something where we should just clamp our heads in horror. . . . In 1900, everybody assumed that masturbation had grave physical consequences; that didn't make it true."

The analogy is fatally flawed. Autoerotic acts differ radically from heteroerotic acts. Masturbation is something the child does for himself; it satisfies one of his biological urges. In that sense, masturbation is similar to urination or defecation. That is why we do not call masturbation a "sexual relationship," a term that implies the involvement of two (or more) persons, one of whom may be an involuntary participant. Masturbation (in private) is an amoral act: strictly speaking, it falls outside the scope of moral considerations. In contrast, every sexual relationship is intrinsically a moral matter; medical (or pseudomedical-psychiatric) considerations ought to play no role in our judgments of such acts. The religiously enlightened person may view same-sex relations as evil. The psychologically enlightened person may view any consensual sex relations as good. Society must decide which sexual acts are permissible, and individuals must decide which sexual acts they condemn, condone, or wish to engage in.

V

The criminal law defines sex between adults and minors as a crime. But the law is a blunt instrument. Technically, an eighteen-year-old male who has a consensual sexual relationship with a seventeen-year-old female is committing a criminal act (statutory rape), even though he might be only one day older than his partner. Such "crimes" generally are not prosecuted.

Sexual contact between a priest and a ten-year-old boy is quite another matter, and here is where the medicalization of unwanted or prohibited behaviors hinders our understanding. To impress the laity, physicians long ago took to using Greek and Latin words to describe diseases. For example, they called inflammation of the lung "pneumonia" and kidney failure "uremia." The result is that people now think that any Greco-Latin word ending in *ia*—or with the suffix *philia* or *phobia*—is a bona fide disease. This credulity would be humorous if it were not tragic.

Bibliophilia means the excessive love of books. It does not mean stealing books from libraries. *Pedophilia* means the excessive (sexual) love of children. It does not mean having sex with them, although that is what people generally have in mind when they use the term. Because children cannot legally consent to anything, an adult using a child as a sexual object is engaging in a wrongful act. Such an act is wrongful because it entails the use of physical coercion, the threat of such coercion, or (what comes to the same thing in a relationship between an adult and a child) the abuse of the adult's status as a trusted authority. The outcome of the act—whether it is beneficial or detrimental for the child—is irrelevant for judging its permissibility.

Saying that a priest who takes sexual advantage of a child entrusted to his care "suffers from pedophilia" implies that there is something wrong with his sexual functioning, just as saying that he suffers from pernicious anemia implies that there something wrong with the functioning of his hematopoietic system. If that were the issue, it would be his problem, not ours. Our problem is that there is something wrong with him as a moral agent. We ought to focus on his immorality and forget about his sexuality.

A priest who has sex with a child commits a grave moral wrong and also violates the criminal law. He does not treat himself as if he has a disease before he is apprehended, and we ought not to treat him that way afterward.

13

Psychiatry's War
on Criminal Responsibility

To renounce the pains and penalties of exhaustive research is to remain a
victim of ill-informed and designing writers, and to authorities that have
worked for ages to build up the vast tradition of conventional mendacity.
—Lord Acton (1834–1902), speech
at the Eranus Society, Cambridge (1897),
quoted in McElrath, *Lord Acton*

I

THE INSANITY PLEA—that is, the assertion of a defendant, typically
charged with murder, that he is not criminally responsible for his offense
because he was insane at the time when he committed the illegal act—is the
oldest and most obvious instance of the medicalization of the law.[1] As formal medical-legal procedures, the insanity defense and civil commitment are
symmetrical tactics: in one case, the idea of mental illness is used to excuse
a guilty person of his crime and incarcerate him in a mental hospital; in the
other, the idea of mental illness is used to incriminate an innocent person as
"dangerously ill" and incarcerate him in a mental hospital. Psychiatry rests
on these two procedures and would disappear in their absence.[2]

I have criticized the medicalizations of the law in previous publications.[3]
In this essay I will present the story of a murder trial where the plea was
insanity. It is an atypical example. When an offender or his lawyer raises
insanity as a defense, the prosecution often does not contest the defendant's
psychiatric claim; instead, in effect it directs the jury to bring in a verdict of
not guilty by reason of insanity and acquiesces in disposing of the defendant by confining him indefinitely in an insane asylum. Alternatively, the

prosecution may contest the defense by asserting that albeit the defendant is mentally ill, his illness is not of sufficient severity to exempt him from the penalties of the criminal law. In the present case, the prosecution pursued a bolder course.

II

In November 1980, Darlin June Cromer, a thirty-four-year-old white woman, was tried in Oakland, California, for the kidnapping and murder of Reginald Williams, a five-year-old African American boy. The charge was "first-degree murder with aggravating circumstances," the aggravating circumstances being racial motives for the killing. Cromer pleaded not guilty by reason of insanity.[4]

The facts about the case were not in dispute. On February 5, 1980, Reginald Williams was abducted from a supermarket. Suspicion quickly pointed to Cromer, known for previous attempts to lure black children into her car and making comments about "killing niggers." When the police visited Cromer, she eagerly confessed luring Reginald into her car, strangling him, and burying his body in a shallow grave on the grounds of a water treatment plant near her home.

Who was Darlin June Cromer? She was a thirty-four-year-old white woman who had spent her entire adult life as a card-carrying mental patient. Diagnosed "schizophrenic" decades earlier, she was in and out of "treatment facilities." In 1980, she was placed on probation for having assaulted a Chinese woman in San Francisco in 1977.

At the trial, three young black children gave vivid testimony about how, the day Williams was killed and also the day before, Cromer tried to entice them into her car. Two refused. One, Steven Willis, accepted Cromer's offer to drive him to his school but saved himself. "After the car passed his school and stopped at an intersection, Willis jumped out and ran several blocks to his school, and told a teacher what had happened."[5]

The prosecution argued that Cromer's motive, as she herself claimed, was racial hatred. Assistant Public Defender Dean Beaupre disagreed. He stated, "There is no question that the defendant did kill this little boy on February 5, 1980. . . . However, this case does not involve racism, it involves insanity. The defendant *is* insane."[6] This was a patent falsehood. If Cromer had been legally insane when Beaupre made his statement, she would not have been on trial: the judge would have had to declare her mentally incompetent to stand trial. What Beaupre was saying, and what four of the most eminent forensic psychiatrists in California were to say in their sworn testimony, was that Cromer was insane in February 1980, some eleven months before she came to trial. Neither Beaupre nor the psychiatrists knew Cromer then; therefore, they could not possibly have had any knowledge about her mental state *at that time*. This contention was the focus of my testimony.

What evidence did the prosecution have for maintaining that Cromer's act was motivated and goal directed, not "meaningless," as newspapers typically characterize murder committed by persons they call "mental patients"? This was some of it:

> In the third day of the trial, a deputy sheriff recounted a free-swinging jail-house conversation she had with Cromer only hours after Cromer's arrest for the murder of Reginald Williams . . . Deputy Dorothy Soto said Cromer "wanted to talk about niggers," and even though Soto didn't encourage her, began a long, rambling diatribe against blacks. Soto, who wrote it all down later, read her recollections to the jury yesterday. She said Cromer sat on a table, talking lucidly. "It is the duty of every white woman to kill a nigger child," Soto quoted Cramer. "I've already killed mine." She said Cromer urged her to kill a black herself.[7]

Beaupre did not put his client on the stand to reject these charges. Instead, he explained that "his client killed because she is consumed by schizophrenic paranoia, not hate for blacks."[8] However, a prison psychologist testified that Cromer told him "she thought the killing of a black child from Alameda would cause a 'snowball' effect in reaction to 'blacks taking over.'"[9]

On February 23, 1981, *Newsweek* ran a feature article on the trial. The reporters characterized Cromer as a "twisted woman," and stated that her attorney, Dean Beaupre, argued that his client was an "acute schizophrenic" who should be acquitted because she was insane:

> "That boy [he told the jury] died because Ms. Cromer was about as psychotic as she could be." . . . Stanford Professor Donald Lunde described her

belief that blacks were like animals, meant to be eaten. "If she isn't crazy,' he concluded, 'who is?'" . . . Prosecutor Albert Meloling . . . tried to make light of what he called "the mystic knights of psychiatry." He imported his own gladiator, maverick psychiatrist and professional debunker Thomas Szasz, who contended that the defendant was "suffering from the consequences of having lived a life badly, stupidly, evilly from the time of her teens."[10]

On January 17, 1981, the jury found Darlin June Cromer guilty of first-degree murder because "she knew what she was doing." She was sentenced to life imprisonment without parole.

Different observers drew different conclusions from this outcome. Dean Beaupre maintained that Cromer was so insane "that she thought she was committing a 'positive act' when she killed the boy." Albert Meloling noted that the jury returned its verdict in a relatively short time and said, "It's obvious that these jurors are saying psychiatrists do not belong in the court room."[11] *Newsweek* conceded that the verdict "will serve one useful purpose: it will keep Darlin June Cromer off the streets for the rest of her life."[12]

III

How did I get involved in the Cromer case? I am not a forensic psychiatrist. I am a critic of psychiatry and especially forensic psychiatry. Ever since the mid-1950s, I have been writing critical essays and books about the role of psychiatry in law. In 1963, *Law, Liberty, and Psychiatry* was published. It was widely and favorably reviewed and became required reading in many law schools. In 1965, *Psychiatric Justice* was published. I continued to publish widely in law review journals. I thus became known in legal circles as a psychiatrist with a principled opposition against both civil commitment and the insanity defense.

In the 1960s and 1970s, I testified in court a few times on behalf of persons incarcerated in mental hospitals trying to regain their liberty. During the same period, I also testified a few times for prosecutors who wished to rebut the plea of "not guilty by reason of insanity." As I have noted earlier, in most such cases—exemplified by the trial of John W. Hinckley Jr.—prosecutor and defense attorney collude, both satisfied with incarcerating the defendant in an insane asylum. The Oakland district attorney, Albert Meloling, was not such a prosecutor. This was a high-profile trial. Meloling was incensed by the deliberate, carefully planned, racially motivated murder of a black boy, especially since the crime was committed in the largely black city of Oakland, California. He was familiar with my views and contacted me. I agreed to testify, provided he was willing to meet one condition: I would not participate in the charade of "examining the patient." Here I must briefly explain why I regard this nonparticipation—which my critics have invariably interpreted as a medical incompetence and irresponsibility or worse—as crucially important for me, both morally and professionally.

Meloling also knew of me because of my behind-the-scenes participation in the prosecution of one of the most sensational mass murders in our times, the 1969 trial of Leslie van Houten, one of the "Manson girls." Van Houten's lawyer called several psychiatrists to testify that she was patently crazy: she believed that Manson was God, carved a large X on her forehead, and committed brutalities that "no sane person could commit." The prosecutor solicited my help. I flew to Los Angeles, discussed the case with him, and suggested that he needed no psychiatric expert on his side at all. There was no need to put me on the stand. Instead, he should concentrate on undermining the credibility of the defense psychiatrists, expose them as quacks always ready to testify that the defendant is not responsible for his crimes and "needs treatment," and rely on the jury's common sense that our basic moral sense demands that such cold-blooded and brutal crimes ought to be punished, and not "excused" by psychiatrists. That is what happened. Leslie van Houten is still in prison. That is the context in which my testimony in the Cromer trial must be viewed.

IV

When a defendant pleads insanity to a charge of murder and when the fact that he committed the murder is not contested, the psychiatric expert is expected to testify about the mental state of the defendant *not* at the time of his examination of the "patient," but at the time when the defendant committed the crime, typically many months before. In the Cromer case, the interval between the crime and the defense psychiatrists' examination of the defendant was approximately ten months.

Psychiatrists regard this practice as medically sound and scientific, and courts and society accept it as similar to expert testimony given by other medical specialists, for example forensic pathologists. I regard the practice as the epitome of junk science and refuse to participate in it. In the first place, there is no objective test for mental illness, as there is for melanoma or pneumonia. What psychiatrists pretentiously call an "examination" is a conversation with the subject and observation of his behavior. The psychiatrist's conclusion is his *opinion* about the subject's mental state *at the time of the examination*. The claim that a psychiatrist is able to determine the mental state of a defendant, say, on January 15, whom he first encounters and examines, say, on November 15, is prima facie absurd. However, our legal-psychiatric system accepts, indeed insists, that this fiction is scientific truth. Few people, and few if any psychiatrists, question this charade. Thus, for a prosecutor who is genuinely determined to prevail against the insanity defense, the best tactic is to unmask the defense psychiatrists as quacks, hired guns masquerading as medical experts. Meloling had no respect for the insanity defense or for psychiatrists always ready to call killers "crazy" and agreed with my suggestion to pursue such a course.

As it turned out, my insistence on *not* examining the defendant and rejecting the option of offering another retroactive diagnosis, different from the diagnosis proffered by the defense experts, proved crucial in convincing the jurors that the defense psychiatrists were deceiving them. The day after the Cromer trial ended, the *San Francisco Chronicle* reported:

> The last witness, called by the prosecution yesterday at a cost of $3,000 was an eminent New York psychiatrist who brought defense lawyers to the edges of their seats when he disputed the previous testimony of four defense experts. . . . Called on rebuttal, Dr. Szasz is author of 17 books, a recognized authority on psychiatry and legal issues and a professor at the State University of New York. He based his testimony on a review of Cromer's extensive medical records. *He added that it would not assist him to examine the defendant.* When asked why by Meloling, Szasz said: "Because I could only determine [what] her mental state is now, not on the day of the murder. That is the nature of psychiatry." The long list of defense

psychiatrists . . . offered a retroactive diagnosis that Cromer was suffering from psychotic delusions.[13]

V

For reasons I shall describe presently, in 1982 the *American Journal of Forensic Psychiatry* reprinted the verbatim transcript of my entire testimony in the Cromer trial. It begins with the so-called direct examination. I am on the witness stand and the prosecutor, Albert Meloling, is questioning me.

> Q. Have you previously testified in the courts in this country on the subject of psychiatric conditions and responsibility?
>
> A. Yes, I have, on a few occasions.
>
> Q. Did you *assist* the District Attorney in Los Angeles County in the case involving one of the Manson Group, that is, the case involving Leslie van Houten?[14]

Like any good lawyer, Meloling asked his witness only questions to which he knew the answer. Note that he used the term "assist" instead of "testify." The defense objected to the question as "irrelevant," the judge sustained the objection, and I did not answer the question. After a brief "voir dire" examination by Dean Beaupre for the defense, Meloling resumed questioning me. After letting me answer questions about how I became familiar with the circumstances of the crime, he continued:

> Q. Now you haven't examined the defendant, have you?
>
> A. No, sir.
>
> Q. Would it assist you in testifying to examine her now?
>
> A. No, sir.
>
> Q. *You understand that what we are concerned with is her mental condition on February 5 of last year?*
>
> A. That is my understanding.
>
> Q. Why would it not help you to examine her now to determine what her mental condition was on February 5, last year?
>
> A. *Because I could only determine by examining her now what her mental condition is now.*

Q. What is the reason for that?

A. That is the nature of a psychiatric examination. I don't know what her mental condition was six months ago. I wouldn't know what it would be six months from now.[15]

Note that this information—elicited from me by the prosecutor for whom I was testifying—was essential for showing the jury that the defense experts had no way of knowing what Cromer's mental condition was at the time of her offense. My crime against psychiatric dogma—namely, not examining the defendant to whom psychiatrists always refer as "patient"— was brought forth and emphasized as part of the prosecution's tactic to secure a conviction. It was not elicited, as is an "admission," by a prosecutor questioning a guilty defendant or a plaintiff's attorney questioning a hostile witness.

Why, then, have psychiatrists and other supporters of psychiatric coercions and excuses ever since accused me of a "failure to examine the defendant" and define my behavior as an "admission" of a wrongdoing? There are three possible answers. One is that my accusers are so convinced of their being in possession of the truth about mental illness that they are deaf to what I say and write. Another possibility is that the critics seize on my deliberate departure from standard forensic-psychiatric practice as evidence, ipso facto, of psychiatric malfeasance. The third possibility is that they hear my message and understand it only too well, and believe that the best defense is an offense and, instead of engaging my argument, slander me.

After a series of other questions, Meloling asked:

Q. You said that the question of whether or not a person was suffering from schizophrenia is really not relevant to the question of whether or not they are responsible?

A. That is correct. . . . Schizophrenics can be and are responsible . . . it is now general practice not to lock them up. So they have all the rights and freedoms of you and me and, therefore, all the responsibilities of you and me to be held responsible for what they do.[16]

After a series of questions intended to clarify for the jury Cromer's reference to blacks as animals, and her wanting to eat her victim, Meloling asked:

Q. You said it is quite common in everyday language to call items by different names?

A. We all do that, all the time, sooner or later we call things by some figure of speech, some so-called metaphor, some other image. I mean if you don't like somebody, you say "You are a son of a bitch." We don't mean that literally he is the son of a bitch. We call somebody "The apple of my eye." We don't mean that you are an apple.

(Laughter)

A. (Continuing) We say to our daughter, "You look so sweet, I can eat you up." That's a figure of speech. The fact that she [Cromer] may have said something like that, *obviously she didn't eat the person,* so a statement she was going to eat it becomes, in my opinion, an outright lie. If she wanted to eat the person, she had plenty of time to eat him.

(Laughter)

(Continuing) And when people use figures of speech, that becomes a matter of speech *for juries to determine, not for psychiatrists.*[17]

Meloling then turned to the issue of Cromer referring to blacks as animals, one psychiatrist claiming that "she was grossly delusional and that her believing things about blacks and Chinese far exceeds simple prejudice."

Q. . . . What is the difference between prejudice and a delusion? Is there a difference?

A. Yes. . . . But obviously this is an utterly subjective and politically and morally loaded question because the idea that blacks are not human or that Jews are not human or that non-Christians, for that matter, are not human, I mean this is what history has been all about, that people see other people as animals, and are ready to kill them. . . . [18]

Finally, Meloling asked the ritually required question of his expert.

Q. You have an opinion as to what Ms. Cromer was suffering from, if anything, on February 5 of this year?

A. Yes, I do.

Q. What is that opinion?

A. That opinion is that she was suffering from the consequences of having lived a life very badly, very stupidly. Very evilly; that from the time of her teens, for reasons which I don't know, she had, whatever she had done, she has done very badly. She was a bad student. There is no evidence that she was a particularly good daughter, sister. She was a bad wife. She was a bad mother. She was a bad employee insofar as she was employable. Then she started to engage [in taking] illegal drugs, then she escalated to illegal assault, and finally she committed this murder. . . . Life is a task. You either cope with it or it gets you . . . If you do not know how to build, you can always destroy. These are the people that destroy us in society, our society, and other people.[19]

Then I was questioned again by Beaupre. He tried to discredit me by arguing that psychiatric diagnoses were just as reliable as medical diagnoses, and my testimony by establishing that I had not read all of the records pertaining to the case, and had been paid $3,000 for my work plus expenses. Meloling didn't let that go unchallenged.

Q. Dr. Szasz, is a psychiatric diagnosis as accurate as a medical diagnosis?

A. Not usually, no.

Q. What is the reason for that?

A. Medical diagnoses deal with objective and demonstrable lesions of the body, broken bones, diseased livers, kidneys, and so on. Psychiatric diagnoses deal with behaviors that human beings display, and they have to be interpreted in moral, cultural, and legal terms and, therefore, different interpreters will arrive at different judgments. . . . Homosexuality was recognized as a mental disease until a few years ago. And now it is no longer a mental disease. . . . but last year, smoking is a disease.

Q. Smoking is now a psychiatric condition?

A. Not condition, sir, a disease.

Q. A disease?

A. A disease. Since January 1980. So is gambling.

Q. Pardon?

A. Gambling is also a disease.

Q. How do you treat that, that is, gambling, do you take away of the money?

(Laughter)

At this point, the judge became so amused by the humor intrinsic to what psychiatrists call a disease, that he answered the question:

Court: You win.

(Laughter)

Witness: That's right. That's my recommendation also.

(Laughter)

Mr. Meloling: I have nothing further.[20]

It was not a good day for the defense. In 1989, the public defender's office appealed Cromer's conviction. "Deputy public defender Colleen Rohann said . . . Cromer had a 20-year history of mental illness and belonged in a psychiatric institution, not a prison."[21] The appeal charged that "Albert Meloling had committed gross misconduct when he called defense psychiatrists 'con men' who were a 'social cancer in society that has to come out.' . . . Cromer had a nearly two-decade history of mental problems and four defense experts said she was insane."[22] The state Supreme Court refused to overturn the murder conviction.

VI

As might be expected, my testimony enraged the psychiatric community. Donald Lunde was one of the most famous and respected forensic psychiatrists in America. My contradicting his expert opinion was an impertinence. Cromer was a certified lunatic. Who could doubt that she was crazy and "belonged" in a mental hospital, not a prison?

Psychiatrists are sore losers. After the trial, they had no trouble—in their own journals and debates—overturning the jury's verdict and, in effect, indicting me of psychiatric malpractice: I didn't examine the "patient," and perhaps worse still, I instilled humor into the proceedings.

Every trial—and surely every sensational murder trial—is theater. It is not possible to understand or appreciate the play without seeing it performed or at least reading the text of it.

Clearly, Lunde viewed the Cromer trial as a duel in which I bested him by foul means. He wrote a letter to the editor of the *American Journal of Forensic Psychiatry,* suggesting publishing the transcript of my testimony accompanied by critical comments by experts in forensic psychiatry. Entitled "The Psychiatrist in Court: People of the State of California v. Darlin June

Cromer," this material was published in the *American Journal of Forensic Psychiatry* in 1982.[23]

The document runs to forty-one pages. I will try to summarize its highlights, in the order in which they appear. In his letter to Ed Miller, the editor of the journal, Lunde suggests that "a reviewer might address . . . the facts that: (1) Dr. Szasz admits [*sic*] that he never examined the defendant, yet renders an opinion about her. (2) Dr. Szasz admits [*sic*] that he did not review all her medical records, yet renders an opinion. (3) Dr. Szasz testifies as an expert in psychiatry that there is no such thing as mental disease."[24]

Note how naturally the language of the KGB agent comes to Lunde's lips. To say that a person *admits* X implies that doing X is immoral, illegal, an affront against legitimate authority. A person does not admit to doing good. We don't say that a person admits that he told the truth; we only say that he admits that he has lied.

I explained already why I regard examining the defendant in such cases and testifying under oath about his mental state many months or years earlier as scientifically contemptible and morally wicked. Regarding Lunde's second charge, that I did not examine *all of her records,* we must keep in mind that Cromer had been a mental patient for more than twenty years. Examining all of her records—assuming that all of them were available, which is doubtful—would probably have taken weeks. Lunde's third charge is, perhaps, the most telling: I am an expert in theology, yet I say there is no God.

The forensic psychiatric establishment decided to rewrite the Cromer case, with the murderer cast as an innocent, sick patient, and I cast as a callous, irresponsible, and wicked psychiatrist. After reviewing the transcript of my testimony, Selwyn M. Smith, MD, professor of psychiatry and psychiatrist-in-chief at Royal Ottawa Hospital, offered this opinion:

> Dr. Thomas Szasz's views are well known . . . disagreements concerning [his] views have been well documented in the psychiatric literature. . . . The preparation by Dr. Szasz prior to giving testimony was in my opinion extremely superficial and *contrary to acceptable standards of practice.* . . . he came to court to testify and in many ways utilized the witness box as a forum for a presentation of his particular views. . . . This flippancy was compounded by his own statement that he saw no need to examine the defendant. Surely

when requested to offer an opinion involving one's expertise as a physician and psychiatrist, one should indeed be prepared to examine the defendant . . . This is particularly true if one is being handsomely paid as was the situation here. I found Dr. Szasz's stance particularly troubling and certainly demeaning to the profession of medicine in general, and psychiatry in particular.[25]

What mattered to Smith was not the truth but the dignity of a psychiatry guilty of charlatanry. As my testimony shows, I said nothing demeaning about medicine. To be sure, I said some unflattering things about psychiatry and the practice of offering psychiatric excuses for murderers in the court room. Smith's comments illustrate that psychiatrists, like other despots, do not tolerate disagreement. If the person who disagrees with them is a mental patient, they punish him with ever more demeaning diagnoses and destructive treatments. If the person is a fellow professional testifying in a court room—where he is safe from the psychiatrists' direct retribution—they punish him by slander and declaring his conduct "unprofessional" and "harmful for patients."

"Dr. Szasz," Smith continued, "is a Professor of Psychiatry, and yet I found his comments pertaining to psychiatry in general and schizophrenia in particular, simplistic, unrealistic, and unscientific. . . . In my opinion, such comments were not helpful to the court. . . . His testimony in general exhibited a poor command of medical-legal principles and *a callous disregard for an ill person*."[26] Smith's remarks are a typical example of psychiatric arrogance. A white person charged with the crime of the racially motivated murder of a black child is here transformed, by psychiatric fiat, into an "ill person" and I am slandered as showing "callous disregard" for the ill. A neat trick, if you can get away with it. Psychiatrists have gotten away with it for the better part of three hundred years, never more successfully than today.

The next contributor to this offensive against me was Joseph C. Finney, LLB, MD, Loyola University Medical Center, Maywood, Illinois. Before I turn to his critique, I want to say a few words about the charge that I inappropriately injected humor into what ought to be a somber proceeding. I am blessed with a good sense of humor and am quite capable, if I want to, of introducing witticism into virtually any verbal communication, spoken or written. However, in this case, laughter in the courtroom began—as the transcript shows—not because I said something witty. Instead, it began when I described how psychiatrists make and unmake diagnoses of mental illnesses, citing smoking and gambling as newly minted diseases. At which point Albert Meloling, the prosecutor, asked me, "How do you treat that, that is, gambling, do you take away the money?" That precipitated laughter in the court room, facilitated by the judge himself breaking out into laughter and volunteering a humorous answer to Meloling's question: "Court: You win." This provoked more laughter. I then answered the question: "That's right. That's my recommendation also," and there was still more laughter. Ridicule is, of course, the most effective weapon against arrogant stupidity. The psychiatrists were not amused.

Interestingly, Dr. Finney based his criticism of my testimony on a psychoanalysis of what he imagined was my personal history. "It may be," he explained, "that the nature of the Cromer crime—murder that was racially motivated—turned Dr. Szasz against the defendant as it turned the prosecutor and the jury. . . . This manifest content [of racial motivation] is irrelevant to the issue of the insanity plea, but it was not irrelevant to Dr. Szasz's willingness to testify. *He specifically associated from killing blacks to killing people of his own ethnic group, thus identifying himself with the victim.*" Finney probably never read a word I wrote and is unaware of my principled opposition against acquitting any defendant on the ground of insanity. To be sure, Finney has managed to discredit me and my testimony with what must be one of the most subtle, yet perhaps persuasive, anti-Semitic comments in contemporary American psychiatric literature.

Finney was a good choice as critical commentator. He did not like what I said and was happy to articulate all his objections. "I find it inappropriate, offensive, and alarming that Dr. Szasz testified that Dr. Lunde's testimony was not only false, but so false as to border on perjury. . . . I am appalled that he said such a thing."[27] Being appalled is not a substitute for showing how or why what I said was untrue. Finney retried the Cromer case in his own mind and, although he had not examined her either, found her not guilty of murder: "I strongly suspect that under our laws, Mrs. Cromer was entitled to be found not guilty by reason of insanity. . . . I conclude that the defense attorney did not do a competent job in defending Mrs. Cromer. . . . He did not cross-examine adequately. . . . I believe an appeal could be taken."[28] An appeal was taken, as I noted earlier, and the verdict of the court was upheld.

A few years ago, when I had occasion to make a study of the life and work of Rudolf Virchow (1821–1902), I came across an episode in his life that closely resembles my refusal to examine Darlin June Cromer.

Virchow, the founder of modern pathology and scientific medicine, was nominally a Protestant but actually an atheist. The publication of his magnum opus, *Cellular Pathology*, in 1858, quickly made him one of most famous medical scientists in the world. "I have dissected thousands of corpses," he declared, "but found no soul in any." He was in the habit of mockingly asking his students engaged in dissection, "Mr. Candidate, have you found a soul already?"[29]

In 1868, Virchow was asked to examine a "patient" and refused. I describe the circumstances and import of this episode in detail in *Pharmacracy*, from which I quote: "In 1868, a Belgian novitiate was supposed to have miraculously survived for three years with 'no sustenance except water and the communion host.' Asked by the Vatican to examine the woman and render an expert medical opinion about the claim, Virchow recognized that there was nothing to examine and refused."[30]

Virchow believed there was no soul that survives the body, or if there is one, it is the concern of miraculous theology, not scientific medicine. He viewed the claim that a young woman lived for three years without food as, prima facie, absurd, if not a deliberate deception. Supposing he undertook to examine the woman in question, what was he supposed to look for?

I see my position regarding the diagnosis of mental illness much the same way. I believe there is no mental illness. No medical examination can detect such a mythical disease. I regard the psychiatrist's claim that he can examine a cold-blooded murderer and detect that, when he committed the crime, he suffered from a mental illness (so severe that it annulled his guilt for his deed), and that his so testifying, under oath, is helping the court by furnishing it with "scientific truth" as a false belief, if not a calculated lie. That the person who utters such an untruth sincerely believes that his lie serves the noble cause of "saving a life" does not alter the fact that it is a deliberate falsehood.

14

Killing as Therapy

The Case of Terri Schiavo

I kept my promise.
                                        —Michael Schiavo, June 2005

Terri didn't die an awful death. I laid a red rose in her hand and said
goodbye.
                                        —Michael Schiavo, September 2005

I

TO WHICH OF HIS PROMISES does Michael Schiavo refer in his inscription on his wife's gravestone? In 1992, during a deposition in his malpractice
suit against the physicians who treated Terri Schiavo for infertility, Michael
was asked how he saw his future with his wife. He replied:

A. I see myself hopefully finishing school and taking care of my wife.

Q. Where do you want to take care of your wife?

A. I want to bring her home.

Q. If you had the resources available to you, if you had the equipment
and the people, would you do that?

A. Yes. I would, in a heartbeat.

Q. How do you feel about being married to Terri now?

A. I feel wonderful. She's my life and I wouldn't trade her for the
world. I believe in my marriage vows.

Q. You believe in your wedding vows, what do you mean by that?

A. I believe in the vows I took with my wife, through sickness, in
health, for richer or poor. I married my wife because I love her and I want
to spend the rest of my life with her.[1]

Michael Schiavo made those statements, under oath, in 1992. In 2005, he had inscribed on Terri's grave marker "February 25, 1990" as the date she had "Departed this Earth."

Are we to interpret Michael Schiavo's self-aggrandizing memorial to refer to his promise of marital fidelity? For more than a decade he has lived with another woman, to whom he refers as his fiancée and with whom he has two children.

Does the marker refer to Michael Schiavo's promise to Terri's parents, Mary and Robert Schindler, that Terri's body would not be cremated and her remains would be buried at a Schindler family plot in Pennsylvania? Two days after she died, Terri was cremated and her ashes were buried at Sylvan Abbey Memorial Park in Clearwater. The Schindlers were notified only after the event.

To what promise keeping, then, does Michael Schiavo refer on his wife's tombstone? Ghoulishly, he brags about his alleged pledge to kill her, in her own best interest. The removal of Terri's feeding tube was, as Joan Didion points out, "repeatedly described as 'honoring her directive.' This, again, was inaccurate: there was no directive. Any expressed wish in this matter existed only in the belated telling of her husband and two of his relatives."[2]

The conflict between the Schindlers and Michael Schiavo was clear. The Schindlers preferred a half-dead daughter above ground to a dead daughter in the grave. Michael preferred a dead ex-wife in the grave to a half-dead wife in a hospice. The Schindlers acknowledged that *they* wanted Terri alive. Michael denied that *he* wanted his wife dead and instead attributed the death wish to Terri's desire to have her life terminated if she were as disabled as she was. This is the fiction the courts upheld.[3] And this is the fiction Michael memorialized—naively and narcissistically—with the inscription he chose to have engraved on Terri's grave marker. "I kept my promise": Sartre could hardly have found a more dramatic example of a husband's bad faith following his wife to her grave.

The Schiavo drama was a classic battle of words: he who controlled the vocabulary controlled the debate and was assured of victory. The Schindlers did not seem to fully recognize this. They failed to emphasize that what Theresa Schiavo allegedly wanted was unconfirmable, based totally on hearsay evidence, and that, in doubtful cases, the long tradition of English and

American law and the Christian religion favors the preservation of life and liberty over their forfeiture. (Michael Schiavo and the Schindlers are Catholics.) The moral default position in the case of Terri Schiavo was clear: she was not dead and killing her was an act of medical killing, a type of heterohomicide. Was it morally justified? In my opinion, it was not: (1) Terri had no living will and there was no credible evidence about what she might have wanted to happen to her half-alive body; (2) Terri's parents wanted to keep her alive, while her husband, living with another woman, wanted her dead; (3) Michael Schiavo's representations lacked credibility and therefore the courts erred in appointing him as Terri's guardian; and (4) assuming that Terri Schiavo would have wanted her life ended, she would not have wanted it ended by being alternately starved and fed, by having her feeding tube repeatedly removed and reinserted over a period of months.

Led by medical ethicists, the mainstream media nevertheless defined the case as a battle between "humanists" and "religious zealots," "rationalists" and "irrationalists." Didion observes, "Yet there remained, on the 'rational' side of the argument, very little acknowledgment that there could be large numbers of people, not all of whom could be categorized as 'fundamentalists' or 'evangelicals,' who were genuinely troubled by the ramifications of viewing a life as inadequate and so deciding to end it. There remained little acknowledgment even that the case was being badly handled."[4]

II

Medicine and science change and, in our day, change rapidly. Fundamental ethical principles are more enduring. Probably the most enduring principle is the injunction against killing human beings, especially when the justification for doing so is morally feeble.

Religion and law decree certain human bonds to be unbreakable, and many people experience them as such. The paradigm of such a bond is that between the pious Jew and his God. Christianity decreed the marriage bond to be similarly unbreakable. This rule, long enshrined in civil law, was repudiated only in recent times.

The principal issue in the Schiavo case—besides the economics of Terri's care—was the conflict between two parties both claiming undying love and loyalty to her: her husband who wanted her dead, and her parents who wanted to keep her alive. In this circumstance, the commandment against killing should alone have been enough to tilt the balance in the parents' favor.

Few moral dilemmas present us with truly novel conundrums. The Schiavo case is not among them. To the contrary, the conflict between the Schindlers and their son-in-law calls to mind the legendary case of the disputed baby in the Old Testament. Two women live together and give birth to babies at about the same time. One baby dies during the night. His mother switches him with the other baby. The living child's mother discovers the deception and brings the dispute to Solomon for arbitration. The Bible tells what happened this way:

> Then came there two women. . . . And the one woman said, O my lord, I and this woman dwell in one house; and I was delivered of a child with her in the house. . . . And this woman's child died in the night; because she overlaid it. And she arose at midnight, and took my son from beside me. . . . and laid it in her bosom, and laid her dead child in my bosom. . . . And the other woman said, Nay; but the living son is my son. . . . Thus they spake before the king. . . . And the king said, Bring me a sword. . . . And the king said, Divide the living child in two, and give half to the one, and half to the other. Then spake the woman whose living child was unto the king . . . O my lord, give her the living child, and in no wise slay it. But the other said, Let it be neither mine nor thine, but divide it. . . . And then the king answered and said, Give her the living child, and in no wise slay it: she is the mother thereof.[5]

Today's Solomon would order both women to undergo psychiatric examination to determine who would make a better mother and would then rule in accordance with the psychiatric "findings," ratified by committees of bioethicists. Herein lies the difference between the language of love and life, and the language of envy and death; between the philosophy of individualism and libertarianism, and the philosophy of collectivism and statism; and between the ethics of justice and the sanctity of life, and the ethics of bioethics and the justification for medical killing.

Solomon, we might be tempted to glibly observe, had it easy because of the second mother's gratuitous comment. Suppose she had said the same thing the first mother said. How would Solomon have decided? We don't know. It would have been a different case, both contending parties choosing life over death. Ironically, Michael Schiavo's conduct reinforces the analogy with the biblical case. In 1993, when he was ostensibly still trying to keep Terri alive, Michael was asked what he had done with Theresa's jewelry. He replied: "Um, I think I took her engagement ring and her . . . what do they call it . . . diamond wedding band and made a ring for myself."⁶ After Terri died, he defined the date of her death as February 25, 1990, and placed that date on his wife's tombstone. If that is when, in Michael Schiavo's view, his wife died, then after that date he considered himself wifeless, a widower who had no morally valid claim to Terri's living body and no legally valid ground for objecting to the Schindlers' desire to assume caring for their daughter who was, de facto and de jure, still alive. I shall abstain here from considering his financial and other possible reasons for not divorcing Terri and fighting the Schindlers' efforts to be her legal guardians.

III

The Schiavo case has generated a vast literature, some in print, much of it on the Internet. Most of this literature analyzes the case from the point of view of the supposed "rights" of the main dramatis personae. What would Terri have wanted had she anticipated her half-alive state? Did feeding and hydration constitute "artificial life support"? Who ought to be her legal guardian? Although the Schindlers' efforts to keep Terri alive received much popular and professional support, most of the debate was straitjacketed into medical terminology and dealt with concepts and issues such as the patient's ability to feel pain, recognize persons, respond to stimuli, permanent vegetative state, brain death, prognosis, rehabilitation, and so forth.

All this was shadowboxing. After more than a decade of being half-dead, it required no sophisticated medical knowledge or technology to conclude that, as a person, Terri Schiavo existed no longer, but that, as a human being, she was still alive. That, after all, is why there had been a long battle about the legitimacy of killing her. She had to be put to death before she could be legally declared dead and her corpse buried or cremated.

Most people who are not religious prefer to be completely dead rather than half-dead. They usually assume that their closest relatives, the persons who truly deserve the awkward appellation "loved ones," share this choice. If they assume otherwise, they are likely to execute a living will expressing their desire to be kept alive as long as possible, regardless of circumstances or costs. The Schindlers themselves wished to keep their daughter alive and believed, with good reason—they were all practicing Catholics—that that is what Terri would have wanted. I shall now briefly examine the Schiavo affair from what I imagine was the Schindlers' point of view, and do so by reference to a classic short story by William Faulkner.

"A Rose for Emily" is a Gothic tale set in a small town in the Old South.[7] Emily Grierson is the only daughter of one of the small town's leading citizens. "The Griersons held themselves a little too high for what they really were. None of the young men were quite good enough for Miss Emily." Mr. Grierson dies, leaving Miss Emily in genteel poverty, living alone in the big house. She becomes a shadowy figure who, however, manages to dominate the town authorities. Afraid to collect the taxes she owes on her home, they are one day confronted with complaints by neighbors about a foul odor emanating from it. "That was two years after her father's death and a short time after her sweetheart—the one we believed would marry her—had deserted her. . . . 'But what will you have me do about it, madam?'," wailed the mayor. "After a week or two the smell went away."

Having set the stage, Faulkner dispels the mystery. A few years after the death of Miss Emily's father, a construction company comes to town, "with riggers and mules and machinery, and a foreman named Homer Barron, a Yankee—a big, dark, ready man, with a big voice and eyes lighter than his face. . . . Presently we began to see him and Miss Emily on Sunday afternoons driving in the yellow-wheeled buggy and the matched team of bays from the livery stable." The construction company leaves and Homer Barron is seen no more. The townsfolk assume that he left with the company.

In fact, rejected by Homer Barron, Miss Emily poisons him with arsenic. The years pass. "Each December we sent her a tax notice, which would be returned by the post office a week later, unclaimed. Now and then we would see her in one of the downstairs windows—she had evidently shut up the top floor of the house . . . Thus she passed from generation to generation—dear, inescapable, impervious, tranquil, and perverse. And so she died."

Distant relatives come to bury her.

> Already we knew that there was one room in that region above stairs which no one had seen in forty years, and which would have to be forced. They waited until Miss Emily was decently in the ground before they opened it. The violence of breaking down the door seemed to fill this room with pervading dust. A thin, acrid pall as of the tomb seemed to lie everywhere upon this room decked and furnished as for a bridal: upon the valance curtains of faded rose color, upon the rose-shaded lights, upon the dressing table, upon the delicate array of crystal and the man's toilet things backed with tarnished silver, silver so tarnished that the monogram was obscured. Among them lay a collar and tie, as if they had just been removed, which, lifted, left upon the surface a pale crescent in the dust. Upon a chair hung the suit, carefully folded; beneath it the two mute shoes and the discarded socks. The man himself lay in the bed. . . . The body had apparently once lain in the attitude of an embrace, but now the long sleep that outlasts love, that conquers even the grimace of love, had cuckolded him. What was left of him, rotted beneath what was left of the nightshirt, had become inextricable from the bed in which he lay; and upon him and upon the pillow beside him lay that even coating of the patient and biding dust. Then we noticed that in the second pillow was the indentation of a head. One of us lifted something from it, and leaning forward, that faint and invisible dust dry and acrid in the nostrils, we saw a long strand of iron-gray hair.

Miss Emily preferred the simulacrum of a husband to no husband at all.[8] The Schindlers preferred the simulacrum of a daughter to no daughter at all. I believe their argument was fatally flawed by their failure to acknowledge this and engaging instead in an ill-considered debate about Terri's medical condition and "prognosis." Their claims that Terri was responsive, that she was not in a vegetative state, and that her prognosis was not hopeless were counterproductive. Watching the case unfold, my impression was that the Schindlers wanted their daughter to be kept alive regardless of how badly damaged and hopeless her condition was. They preferred a daughter half-dead or four-fifths dead to no daughter at all. But they never said so. Nor did they offer to foot the bill for caring for Terri.

There is no evidence, in the many documents I have seen, that the Schindlers ever offered to pay for Terri's care. Either they did not have the means to do so or did not want to expend their funds in that way. Exploring the economic aspects of the cost of caring indefinitely for persons in Terri's condition would require another essay or, rather, a substantial monograph. Let me say only that I surmise—and I believe it is reasonable to surmise—that had the Schindlers been billionaires, they would have mounted a very different legal challenge against their alienated and angry son-in-law: they could have petitioned the courts—in a type of habeas corpus plea—for the opportunity to care for Terri, indefinitely and at no cost to the public, supported by appropriate medical, nursing, and other help. I believe the courts would have found this request difficult to reject.

IV

Let me now say a few words about the moral dilemmas of medical killing, with special reference to personal autonomy, the prohibition of suicide, and the war on drugs. I have written extensively about these subjects and a few observations about them must suffice here. The Schiavo case touches on many of the difficult economic, moral, legal, and social dilemmas that the combination of advances in modern medical technology and the national socialization of heath care services present to advanced Western societies. (I use the term "national socialism" in its precise descriptive sense, to refer to state control of important sectors of the nation's economy, not to the German Nazi regime.) Unwilling to tackle these problems, the judicial authorities in Florida sidestepped them and chose to pretend that the conflict between husband and parents ought to be decided on the basis of a fictitious autonomy they attributed to Terri.

Autonomy is self-government. It can be curtailed only by the self and the state. We limit our own autonomy every time we make a promise or enter into a contract, for example by marrying. The state limits our autonomy every time it prohibits an act, especially the type of act that John Stuart Mill aptly called "self-regarding," such as self-medication. Our autonomy is now strictly limited by a political system I call the therapeutic state.[9] Paradoxically, when I was growing up in a not-very-democratic Hungary and the world was on the verge of a totalitarian nightmare, personal autonomy was less limited. No one tried to prevent individuals—not even school children—from killing themselves. Opiates and sleeping pills were widely available and their possession was not prohibited. Although traditionally a Roman Catholic country, Hungary has long had, and still has, the highest suicide rate in the world.

"The free man owns himself. He can damage himself with either eating or drinking; he can ruin himself with gambling. If he does he is certainly a damn fool, and he might possibly be a damned soul; but if he may not, he is not a free man any more than a dog."[10] The words are Gilbert K. Chesterton's. He was a devout Catholic and a passionate conservative, not a liberal, much less a libertarian. Today, with the whole "civilized" world waging wars on drugs and suicide, few people agree with this statement.

Physicians, especially psychiatrists, have been waging war on autonomy for more than 200 years. As medical professionals acquired more knowledge about the human body and its diseases, they sought increasing control over it. Physicians attacked autonomy along three fronts, corresponding to three basic human urges—sex, drugs, and death. Supported by pseudoscience and the state, they declared self-abuse, self-medication, and self-killing diseases and punished them as offenses against the public health and hence the public good. The free man owns himself. The therapeutic state prohibits self-ownership.

Terri Schiavo had no right to kill herself when she was fully alive. "Suicidality," defined as a "symptom of depression," is the main justification for civil commitment—an act of depriving a person not only of autonomy but of liberty. Nevertheless, so the story goes, Terri Schiavo had a right to have her life terminated when she was only half-alive because, allegedly, that is what she would have wanted had she been able to express her wants. We often believe X not because X is true, but because believing X helps us to achieve our selfish purposes. We have no right to suicide, yet we insist that respect for "patient autonomy" requires that we have a right to physician-assisted suicide.[11]

Reconsider the basic facts of the case. For fifteen years, Terri Schiavo's half-alive body lay in bed. Ostensibly, during all this time, both her husband and her parents wanted to "help" her. Initially, they helped her to stay alive.

No one then spoke of Terri's wish to be killed. Then came a sudden reversal, when Michael "remembered" Terri's alleged verbal living will. Michael now sought to help Terri by ending her life as soon as possible, while the Schindlers helped her by preserving her life as long as possible. At the same time—characteristically for the times we live in—neither party was willing to assume real obligation to care for her; both parties wanted to use the power and purse of the state to implement their wishes. Michael wanted the state to end Terri's life. The Schindlers wanted the state to keep Terri alive and pay for her care. (Only a small, initial part of Terri's care was paid by the malpractice insurance money awarded to Michael. By the end, the taxpayer was paying the bills.)

V

The truth is that the Schiavo case had nothing whatever to do with what we fatuously call "patient autonomy." Instead, it had to do with property rights and money—specifically, with deciding, first, who was the rightful "owner" of Terri's half-alive body, and second, who was to pay for keeping her alive till she was pronounced legally dead.

Regardless of the medical-technical term we choose to describe Terri's state—coma, permanent vegetative state, severe and irreversible brain damage—two things are clear: that before her feeding tube was removed, she was not dead; and that she was helpless and dependent on others for survival in much the same way that a newborn baby is: she could breathe and metabolize food, but needed to be fed, and hydrated, and cared for. The difference between Terri and a baby was that Terri was destined to remain totally disabled and dependent until she died.

There is nothing unusual or uncommon about this sort of situation. On the contrary, the problem is pervasive and perennial. But we must be clear about whose problem it is and what the true nature of the problem is. The problem is not the patient's, just as the problem of abortion is not the fetus's. Terri *had* no problem. She *was* the problem. For whom? For her husband, for her parents, and for the agents of society charged with protecting certain classes of dependents. Under the age-old legal principle of *parens patriae*, incompetent human beings needing and deserving care and protection were, in John Locke's words, "idiots, infants, and the insane." Today, in addition to "idiots, infants, and the insane," the category of such incompetents includes the aged, the unconscious, and persons, like Terri, in a chronic vegetative state.

If relations among family members are harmonious and some are willing to care for a disabled person, they do so, and that is the end of the matter. Many parents care for their severely handicapped children, and many adult children care for their demented parents. If the persons responsible for the dependent are wealthy, they typically delegate the task to others. That is the way Joseph Kennedy Sr. cared for his daughter Rosemary after the lobotomy to which he subjected her rendered her, too, only half a person. Severely brain damaged, Rosemary was sent to a Catholic convent home in Wisconsin, lavishly endowed by Kennedy to conceal his embarrassing deed and care for his damaged daughter. Out of sight and out of mind, Rosemary "lived" there for more than sixty years, until her death in 2005 at the age eighty-six.

Family members may also agree on the opposite course, which they often do in the kind of hopeless situation with which Terri's husband and parents were faced. They then instruct medical personnel to desist from heroic measures to prolong the dying process. This is one of the functions of hospice care. It is important to emphasize in this connection that Terri Schiavo did not properly qualify for such care. Move to a hospice facility requires that the attending physician certify that the patient has only six months to live and that the patient or guardian relinquish all treatment other than that for pain.[12]

In the Schiavo controversy, the courts upheld the fiction that Terri's autonomy required that she be medically killed, in her own best interest. In view of the fact that we live in a country whose laws prohibit suicide and often deny patients with terminal illnesses the painkillers they need, the doctors' and courts' sensitivities to patient autonomy were, in this case, touching to say the least. Michael requested the court to attribute to Terri the legally enforceable right to physician-assisted suicide. That this decision favored Michael's personal and financial interests, and the taxpayers' economic interests, was purely coincidental.

The Schiavo case—like Shakespeare's *Lear* or *Hamlet*—was and remains great drama. It holds up a mirror, as it were, that reflects our selfishness in conflict with our attachments, our moral uncertainties and vanities, and, above all else, our boundless hypocrisies about drugs, dying, and medical care.

Enlisting physicians in the task of killing people, whether patients or enemies of the state, is not a new idea. The fact that the Hippocratic oath prohibits medical killing suggests that physicians and their superiors must have found it a temptation. The practice seems to have started in Rome under Nero, who would send "doctors to those who hesitated to execute his order to commit suicide, . . . instruct[ing] them to 'treat' (*curare*) the victims, for thus the lethal incision was called."[13] The guillotine and the gas chamber were developed by medical doctors. The Nazi medical Holocaust was an unabashed euthanasia program planned and carried out by physicians.

In English literature, the first reference to death as treatment appears in Thomas More's *Utopia* (1516). He wrote, "Should life become unbearable for these incurables, the magistrates and priests do not hesitate to prescribe euthanasia. . . . When the sick have been persuaded of this, they end their lives willingly either by starvation or drugs."[14]

The practice of routinely referring to the ostensible beneficiary of physician-assisted suicide (PAS) as a "patient," albeit seemingly harmless, prejudges the act as medical and legitimizes it as beneficial ("therapeutic"). To be sure, a person dying of a terminal illness is, ipso facto, considered a patient. However, *dying is not a disease;* it may, inter alia, be a consequence of disease (or other causes, such as accident or violence). More importantly, *killing* (oneself or someone else) is not, and by definition cannot be, a *treatment.*

Strictly speaking, the phrase "assisted suicide" is an oxymoron. Suicide is killing oneself. We ought to call it autohomicide, to distinguish it from heterohomicide, which is the correct name of the act by which Terri Schiavo's life was terminated. Neither autohomicide nor heterohomicide is *a medical matter.* Both are *legal, moral, economic, and political matters.*[15]

A person has no *need* for another to perform a service that he could perform for himself, provided, of course, that he wants to and is allowed to perform the service. If a person knows how to drive but prefers to be driven by someone else, he has no *need* for a chauffeur, he *wants* a chauffeur. Such a person is not receiving "chauffeur-assisted driving." The same is true for killing oneself.

Let us not forget that physicians have always been partly agents of the state and are now in the process of becoming de facto government employees. Therefore, unless a person kills himself, we cannot be certain that his death is voluntary; under no circumstances should such a death be called "suicide." If a person is physically unable to kill himself and someone else kills him, then we are dealing with a clear case of heterohomicide (euthanasia, mercy killing, or medical murder, as the case may be). Moreover, if a physician carries out the act, which is what happened in the Schiavo case, then we cannot be sure that the patient did not want to change his mind in the last moment, but could not or was not allowed to do so. We know that many persons who prepare advance directives requesting that physicians abstain from "heroic measures" to prolong their dying change their minds when the time comes to honor their own prior requests.

In short, conjoining the terms "assisted" and "suicide" is cognitively misleading and politically mischievous. The term "physician-assisted suicide" is a euphemism, similar to terms like "pro-choice" (for abortion) and "right to life" (for prohibiting abortion). We ought to reject PAS not only as social policy but also as a conventionally used phrase, especially so long as suicide remains illegal, prohibited by mental health law and punished by psychiatric agents of the state.

Words are important. We must be careful about what we call the persons who receive and deliver suicide-assistance services. If we call the persons who receive the services "patients" and those who deliver them "physicians," then dying by means of such a service is, ipso facto, a "treatment," and PAS becomes an approved cause of death, like dying from a disease. In short, the legal definition of PAS as a procedure that only a physician can perform expands the medicalization of everyday life, extends medical control over personal conduct, especially at the end of life, and diminishes patient autonomy.

VI

Let us call a spade a spade. Terri Schiavo was killed: to be precise, she was executed, in accordance with a legally valid court order, by starvation and dehydration. Why? Because no one—not her husband, not her parents, not any philanthropist, not the American taxpayer—was willing to pay to keep her alive. The elephant in the room no one wanted to see was money. Had Terri's parents been Melinda and Bill Gates, and had they wanted to keep Terri alive, there would have been no "case." If we believe that executing innocent people is wrong, then the Schiavo case presents no ethical problem. It presents economic, political, and social problems.

Millions of persons all over the world—infants, old people, severely disabled persons—would die if they were not given food and water by others. Tens of thousands of persons, whose quality of life is not measurably better than Terri Schiavo's was, languish in nursing homes, tied to wheelchairs and drugged with Haldol. Looking after them for seven years, how many of their relatives could "remember" that the "patients" chose to die when they fell into such a state? How many could produce "credible witnesses" from among siblings or close friends to testify that they heard the patients say that? Would this be sufficient legal ground to starve them to death?

The problem is obvious: dependency. Formerly, this was a problem for the family and the church. Now, it is a problem for the state. Why? Because the modern national-socialist state has assumed the social-economic functions of the church and is assuming more and more of the social-economic functions of the family.

Sir William Osler (1849–1919), perhaps the most celebrated physician in the history of American medicine, foresaw the problem of mass dependency in mass society and boldly offered a notorious recommendation. In 1905, Osler resigned from John Hopkins Medical School, of which he had been a founder, to accept the even more prestigious position of Regius Professor of Medicine at Oxford. Nearly fifty-six years old, contemplating his own aging, he delivered an address titled "The Fixed Period," declaring that "men over the age of sixty were useless," that "the history of the world shows that a very large proportion of the evils may be traced to sexagenarians," and that "peaceful departure by chloroform might lead to incalculable benefits," for them as well as for society.[16] Subsequently, Osler said, not very persuasively, that his proposal was "whimsical." However, many people took it seriously. His supposed spoof had temporarily enriched the language, generating the verb "Oslerize" (meaning "euthanize"), used both in jest and in earnest.

When Osler delivered his speech, he was a revered figure in American medicine. Nevertheless, the press—then still vigilant about protecting personal freedom from medical statism—was alarmed. An editorial in the *New York Times* castigated his remarks and compared his proposal to the practices of "savage tribes . . . whose custom it is to knock their elders on the head whenever the juniors find their elders in their own way."[17] Two days after the address was denounced in the papers, a Civil War veteran shot himself to death. A clipping of Osler's address was found on his desk. The story was front-page news in a report entitled "Suicide Had Osler Speech." Undaunted, Osler angrily retorted, "I meant just what I said, but it's disgraceful, this fuss that the newspapers are making about it." In his hagiography of Osler, Harvey Cushing, the famed Harvard neurosurgeon, stated, "Efforts were made in vain to get him to refute his statement; and though there can be no question that he was sorely hurt, he went on his way with a smile."[18]

His later disclaimers notwithstanding, Osler was serious. This conclusion is supported by his favorable reference to John Donne's now forgotten defense of suicide in *Biathanatos* (1646),[19] and also by the fact that Osler's essay and title were inspired by Anthony Trollope's (1815–1882) novel, also titled *The Fixed Period*. Trollope's tale, cast in the mold of a futuristic utopia/dystopia, takes place on the imaginary island "Britanulla," where the human life span is fixed at sixty-five years.[20] At the end of their sixty-sixth year, men and women are admitted to a college for a twelve-month period of preparation for euthanasia by chloroform. Trollope was sixty-seven when he wrote the novel. A year later he died, without benefit of chloroform. Despite his stature as the giant of American medicine, Osler never lived down his flirtation with medical killing.

VII

Like nearly everyone in America today, Michael Schiavo too has become an expert on medical ethics. On September 24, 2005, he traveled to the Twin Cities to speak at a conference on medical ethics honoring Dr. Ronald Cranford, a Minneapolis neurologist who served as his medical advisor during the debacle. Michael declared, "I never, in my entire life, thought I would be thrown into such a national debate. . . . All I wanted to do was carry out my wife's wishes. . . . Terri didn't die an awful death, . . . As she died, I laid a red rose in her hand and said goodbye."[21] His address was met by a standing ovation from the more than 200 people in attendance.

Writing after the hurricane Katrina in August 2005, universal expert Thomas Friedman opines, "There is something troublingly self-indulgent and slothful about America today—something that Katrina highlighted and that people who live in countries where the laws of gravity still apply really noticed. . . . We let the families of the victims of 9/11 redesign our intelligence organizations, and our president and Congress held a midnight session about the health care of one woman, Terri Schiavo, while ignoring the health crisis of 40 million uninsured."[22]

Professing compassion for the masses, Friedman, the true Jacobin, self-righteously dismisses the rights of the individual. In a different yet similar context, Edmund Burke (1729–1797) alluded to Rousseau in this priceless portrait of the modern totalitarian-humanist:

> Benevolence to the whole species, and want of feeling for every individual with whom the professors come in contact, form the character of the new philosophy. . . . He melts with tenderness for those only who touch him by the remotest relation, and then, without one natural pang, casts away, as a sort offal and excrement, the spawn of his own disgustful amours, and sends his children to the hospital of foundlings. The bear loves, licks, and forms her young; but bears are not philosophers. Vanity, however, finds its account in reversing the train of our natural feelings. Thousands admire the sentimental writer; the affectionate father is hardly known in his parish. . . . As the relation between parents and children is the first among the elements of vulgar, natural morality, they erect statues to a wild, ferocious, low-minded, hard-hearted father, of fine general feelings—a lover of his kind, but a hater of his kindred.[23]

Vanity, indeed. In 1993, while ostensibly trying to keep his wife Terri alive, Michael Schiavo converts her engagement ring and wedding band into a ring for himself; in June 2005, after Terri is cremated and her ashes are buried, he defines the date of her death as February 25, 1990, and uses her gravestone as a placard for congratulating himself on his self-proclaimed moral fidelity to her; and now, while continuing to loudly disclaim interest in publicity, he lectures on medical ethics.

Michael Schiavo had a choice to relinquish the care of his half-dead wife to her parents, who were begging him to let them assume that role, and could have avoided the ensuing publicity that he claims he abhorred. He refused to do so. Cui bono?

15

Peter Singer's Ethics of Medicalization

"We prefer to do things comfortably" [said Mustapha Mond, the Controller].

"But I don't want comfort. I want God, I want poetry, I want real danger, I want freedom, I want goodness, I want sin."

"In fact," said Mustapha Mond, "you're claiming the right to be unhappy."

"All right, then," said the Savage defiantly, "I'm claiming the right to be unhappy."

—Aldous Huxley, *Brave New World* (1932)

I

PETER SINGER (1946–) is the Ira W. DeCamp Professor of Bioethics at Princeton University and laureate professor at the Centre for Applied Philosophy and Public Ethics, University of Melbourne, Australia. Why do I consider his views—which I think are mistaken and wicked—in this volume? I do so because he is a prominent figure in contemporary bioethics and because his "preference utilitarian perspective" is a striking example of the contemporary debauchment of morality and politics by means of the medicalization of ethics. In his "Philosophical Self-Portrait," a summary of his principal contentions, Singer writes:

> I am probably best known for *Animal Liberation* (1975, 1990), a book that gave its title to a worldwide movement. The essential philosophical view it maintains is simple but revolutionary. Species is, in itself, as irrelevant to moral status as race or sex. Hence all beings with interests are entitled

134

to equal consideration: that is, we should not give their interests any less consideration than we give to the similar interests of members of our own species. Taken seriously, this conclusion requires radical changes in almost every interaction we have with animals, including our diet, our economy, and our relations with the natural environment.[1]

Singer's views are neither as novel nor as secular as he thinks they are. His brand of utilitarianism is a hodgepodge of sentimental Schweitzerian "reverence for life," brutal quasi-Nazi eugenicism, Marxist anticapitalism, and therapeutic statism, wrapped in the rhetoric of *épater les bourgeois* (astound the conventional man). Singer calls his system "practical ethics." In fact, nothing could be more impractical:

> I approach each issue by seeking the solution that has the best consequences for all affected. By "best consequences," I understand that which satisfies the most preferences, weighted in accordance with the strength of the preferences. Thus my ethical position is a form of preference-utilitarianism. . . . I apply this ethic to such issues as equality (both between humans, and between humans and non-human animals), abortion, euthanasia and infanticide, the obligations of the wealthy to those who are living in poverty, the refugee question, our interactions with non-human beings and ecological systems, and obedience to the law. A non-speciesist and consequentialist approach to these issues leads to striking conclusions. It offers a clear-cut account of why abortion is ethically justifiable, and an equally clear condemnation of our failure to share our wealth with people who are in desperate need. . . . Perhaps it is only to be expected, though, that there should be heated opposition to an ethic that challenges the hitherto generally accepted ethical superiority of human beings, and the traditional view of the sanctity of human life.[2]

Singer is a disciple of the English utilitarian philosopher Jeremy Bentham (1748–1832), who argued that the right action was that which would cause "the greatest happiness of the greatest number." Singer uses this vacuous principle as the basis for what he calls "preference-utilitarianism." His ethical reasoning, if one may call it that, depends heavily on the use of postulating improbable analogies and treating them as identities. Virtue, personal responsibility, individual liberty, decency, honesty, loyalty, and kindness are terms notably absent from Singer's moral discourse. His academic standing is a symptom of the moral impoverishment of our academia.

II

With a seemingly straight face Singer asks, "Can a non human animal be a person?" and answers, "It sounds odd to call an animal a person. This oddness may be no more than a symptom of our habit of keeping our own species sharply separated from others."[3] Singer's insistence that a nonhuman animal may be a person is no more than a symptom of his desire to raise animals that can experience suffering to the moral status of persons and hence not killable, and lower persons who cannot experience suffering to the status of nonpersons and hence killable.

Singer links his claim that some animals have a right to life with the claim that some humans do not: "It is certainly true that the traditional view that life should be respected simply because it is human is one that I reject. . . . I don't believe that a newborn infant has a right to life. . . . We ought to question something that we ordinarily take for granted, the idea that it is always wrong to take the life of an innocent human being."[4] In other words, Singer wants to abolish the old rule that killing innocent humans is wrong, and replace it with the new rule that it is wrong only if the subject possesses certain cognitive capacities. In *Practical Ethics*, Singer formulates this principle as follows:

> [T]he fact that a being is a human being, in the sense of a member of the species Homo sapiens, is not relevant to the wrongness of killing it; it is rather characteristics like rationality, autonomy, and self-consciousness that make a difference. Infants lack these characteristics. Killing them, therefore, cannot be equated with killing normal human beings, or any other self-conscious being. This conclusion is not limited to infants who, because of irreversible intellectual disabilities, will never be rational, self-conscious beings.[5]

Many mental health professionals believe that certain mental patients meet Singer's criteria for not being fully human and would therefore qualify as nonpersons.

The proposition that an innocent human being has a right not to be killed only if he knows he is alive and can see himself as existing over time is more troublesome than Singer allows. That principle would justify killing not only infants, idiots, and the insane—the traditional triad of persons categorized as not fully human by English and American law—but also persons in a permanent or temporary coma, persons under anesthesia, and even persons soundly asleep. After all, a person in deep, dreamless sleep does not know that he is alive and cannot see himself as existing over time. The fact that he will wake up and meet Singer's criteria for having a right to life does not count: the difference between a sleeper's awakening to self-consciousness and an infant's achieving that state is a matter of time—one takes a few minutes or hours, the other a few months or years.

Singer's reasoning to justify infanticide comes across as heartless and unfeeling. He writes, "I shall assume that the parents do not want the disabled child to live." But killing a child [*sic*], even a physically imperfect one, is not a private act, like bathing him or her. It is a quintessentially public, political act. In a government under law, killing is made permissible or impermissible by law. The parents' wishes are irrelevant. Not according to Singer's utilitarian calculation: regarding the permissibility of killing an infant simply because he suffers from hemophilia, he writes, "The total view makes it necessary to ask whether the death of the hemophiliac infant would lead to the creation of another being who would not otherwise have existed. In other words, if the hemophiliac child is killed, will his parents have another child? If they would, is the second child likely to have a better life than the one killed?"[6]

Singer the "consequentialist" does not tell us who would or should be legally authorized to kill such infants. Parents? Physicians? Professional executioners? Who would own the remains of such infants? To what use could they be put? The mind boggles.

III

In addition to advocating killing abnormal babies and normal infants unwanted by their parents, Singer also advocates two kinds of medical killings, "voluntary euthanasia" (VE) and "physician-assisted suicide" (PAS).

He writes, "It is therefore odd that those who have claimed to be defenders of individual rights and freedom have not all come to the support of the legalization of voluntary euthanasia."[7] Singer supports the *physician's right* to administer VE and PAS, but does not support the *individual's right* to commit suicide. The following remarks illustrate Singer's ambivalence about personal autonomy: "Do these arguments for voluntary euthanasia perhaps give too much weight to individual freedom and autonomy? After all, we do not allow people free choice on matters like, for instance, the taking of heroin. This is a restriction of freedom but, in the view of many, one that can be justified on paternalistic grounds. If preventing people from becoming heroin addicts is *justifiable* paternalism, why isn't preventing people from having themselves killed?"[8] Why, indeed? What restriction of personal autonomy is *unjustifiable paternalism*? Note that Singer asks why it isn't justifiable paternalism to prevent "people from having themselves killed." He does not consider the option of abstaining from forcibly preventing people from killing themselves.

Clearly, the fundamental Anglo-American political concept of the rule of law plays virtually no role in Singer's political philosophy. As Gary L. Francione, distinguished professor of law at Rutgers University School of Law, notes:

> Singer's theory does not concern rights since Singer does not believe that animals or humans have rights. Indeed, Singer himself refers to his theory as one of "animal liberation" and states that claims of right are "irrelevant." . . . It is easy to understand why Singer rejects rights in light of his view that only the consequences (understood in terms of the preference satisfaction of those affected) of acts matter. A right is generally regarded as "a moral trump card that cannot be disputed." A right serves as a type of protection that cannot be sacrificed even if the consequences of doing so would be very desirable.[9]

Similarly, a right guarantees that, in a free society, any act not prohibited by law is, ipso facto, permitted. Although the act may be wicked, it is not illegal. For example, in 1932 the law prohibited people from selling liquor to other people at their request. Now the law prohibits people from killing other people at their request (VE). Alcohol was *not legalized* in 1933.

Prohibition was *repealed*. Properly posed, the questions about suicide are: Should we repeal the presently enforced psychiatric prohibition against suicide? Should we permit a person to hire a physician to kill him? Should we make such killing permissible only by physicians? Only under conditions defined and determined by doctors? In short, should we make voluntary death available by prescription only, much as we make the voluntary use of effective painkillers available by prescription only?

Suicide, let us remember, involves only one person in the act of terminating his own life (autohomicide), whereas killing another person involves two or more persons in the act of terminating another person's life (heterohomicide). They are radically different acts.[10]

I V

Let us return to Singer's views on PAS. He writes: "He ["suicide doctor" Jack Kevorkian] helps people who are terminally ill and don't want to go on to the end."[11] This is false. In his book *Prescription: Medicide*, Kevorkian states, "Help[ing] suffering or doomed persons to kill themselves . . . is merely . . . [a] distasteful professional obligation . . . What I find most satisfying is the prospect of making possible the performance of invaluable experiments or other beneficial acts."[12]

Singer calls the persons Kevorkian killed "people." Kevorkian calls them "patients." Kevorkian had no license to practice medicine, and the people he "helped" did not come to him to be diagnosed or treated. They traveled, sometimes thousands of miles, to secure his services as medical killer. If they could do that, they could have killed themselves by other means, for example by architect-assisted suicide, aka jumping off a tall building. They came to Kevorkian, then, either to obtain lethal drugs to which they had no access but Kevorkian did, albeit illegally; or they came to die by Kevorkian's hands rather than their own, anxious to depict medical killing as "therapy." Kevorkian was eager to oblige, portraying himself as a heroic fighter for a "right to suicide."

The so-called problem of physician-assisted suicide thus comes down to the question: Why do people need the help of doctors to kill themselves? The answer is because selling and buying lethal drugs is illegal; because physicians (and pharmacists) have privileged access to such drugs and can, under certain conditions, dispense them to persons deemed to be patients; and because individuals who try to kill themselves but fail—that is, who attempt to commit "physician-unassisted suicide"—are punished by psychiatric imprisonment and torture. Singer does not consider, much less condemn, coercive psychiatric suicide-prevention principles and practices.

Indeed, it is fair to say that he nowhere criticizes the idea of mental illness or the incarceration of the mentally ill. He writes, "What, for instance, of those we call 'psychopaths'? . . . Psychopaths are certainly abnormal, but whether it is proper to say they are mentally ill is another matter." Another matter? Ordinarily, Singer accepts people's self-evaluation of their happiness or lack of it. "Psychopaths," whoever they are, are an exception: "Must we accept psychopaths' own evaluation of their happiness? They are, after all, notoriously persuasive liars. Moreover, even if they are telling the truth as they see it, are they qualified to say that they are really happy . . . ?"[13]

In the past, church and state regulated suicide. Today, medicine and the state regulate it. Singer likes it that way and wants to expand the power of the therapeutic state: *"If acts of euthanasia could only be carried out by a member of the medical profession, with the concurrence of a second doctor, it is not likely that the propensity to kill would spread unchecked throughout the community."*[14] Three of Singer's grandparents died in the Holocaust. Nazi medical killing was carried out by members of the medical profession, with the concurrence of many more than two doctors approving it.

Death control or ending one's own life because that is what one wants is a personal matter. If we treat suicide as a medical matter, dispensing it by prescription, we do not give control to the person who wants to kill himself; we give it to the state and its medical agents. We have been through the same process with pain control: giving patients access to effective pain medication by prescription does not give them control over ending their pain; it gives control to the state and its medical agents. "Liberty," declared Acton, "is the prevention of control by others." Either the state controls the means for suicide and thus deprives persons of a fundamental right to self-determination, or we control it and assume responsibility for the manner of our own death. Giving physician-agents of the state the power to prevent suicide by psychiatric coercion and the power to provide "suicide" by medical prescription does not enhance patient autonomy, as Singer claims. It enhances the prestige and power of the state and its bureaucratic agents.

V

Singer, it must be acknowledged, is willing to carry his argument to its logical conclusion, regardless of how bizarre the result. Under the heading "Some facts about poverty," he states, "In the discussion of euthanasia in Chapter 7, we questioned the distinction between killing and allowing to die, concluding that it is of no intrinsic ethical significance."[15] The assertion that there is no "intrinsic ethical significance" between killing and allowing to die—one an act of commission, the other an act of omission (at worse)—is an opinion, not a fact, and an odious opinion at that. "If these"—that is, the identity between omission and commission—"are the *facts*," Singer continues, "we cannot avoid concluding that by not giving more than we do, people in rich countries are allowing those in poor countries to suffer from absolute poverty, with consequent malnutrition, ill health, and death. This is not a conclusion that applies only to governments. It applies to each absolutely affluent individual."[16] Is Singer an "absolutely affluent individual"? Yes. Does he follow his own precept? No.

In an interview in *Reason* magazine, Singer restates his view "that the affluent in developed countries are killing people by not giving away to the poor all of their wealth in excess of their needs." The interviewer continues:

> How did he come to this conclusion? "If allowing someone to die is not intrinsically different from killing someone, it would seem that we are all murderers." . . . He calculates that the average American household needs $30,000 per year; to avoid murder, anything over that should be given away to the poor. "So a household making $100,000 could cut a yearly check for $70,000." . . . Singer's proclamation about income has also come back to haunt him. To all appearances, he lives on far more than $30,000 a year. Aside from the Manhattan apartment—he asked me not to give the address or describe it as a condition of granting an interview—he and his wife Renata . . . have a house in Princeton. The average salary of a full professor at Princeton runs around $100,000 per year; Singer also draws income from a trust fund that his father set up and from the sales of his books. . . . he is certainly

living on a sum far beyond $30,000. When asked about this, he forthrightly admitted that he was not living up to his own standards. . . . [He] hinted that he would increase his giving when everybody else started contributing similar amounts of their incomes. There is some question as to how seriously one should take the dictates of a person who himself cannot live up to them.[17]

The jet-setting Singer—a frequent lecturer who receives $15,000 per performance—masquerades as an ascetic.[18] Not surprisingly, he emphasizes that "[c]onsequentialists start not with moral rules but with goals. They assess actions by the extent to which they further these goals." Rules are objective and observable, goals are neither. Would Singer, the "preference utilitarian," prefer that driving be regulated not by traffic rules but by the goal of safe travel?

Singer does not say whether the ethics of his consequentialism rests on *goals as intentions avowed by the actor* or the *actual consequences of the actor's actions as observed and judged by others.* Characteristically, he regards foreign aid as a measure that, a priori, ameliorates pauperism. This is contrary to the evidence, which is that it aggravates it. "Money gifts save the poor man who gets them, but give longer life to pauperism in the country,"[19] warned Lord Acton.

Social policies have two kinds of consequences: intended and unintended. The intended consequences are always virtuous; the unintended consequences are all too often wicked. Singer ignores or is ignorant of the vast literature on this subject, particularly that which demonstrates the disastrous consequences of foreign aid. . . . "Money gifts save the poor man who gets them, but give longer life to pauperism in the country." More recently, Lord Bauer's empirical studies demonstrated that aid increased the patronage and power of the recipient governments, which often pursued policies that stifled entrepreneurship and market forces. He memorably defined foreign aid as "an excellent method for transferring money from poor people in rich countries to rich people in poor countries."[20]

Regarding wealth and poverty, Singer's ignorance is unlimited and invincible. He disregards that the primary source of wealth is work. Because it is better to be rich than poor, poverty has always excited compassion and riches the suspicion of wrongdoing. The inchoate belief that being wealthy is somehow shameful or sinful has a long history, probably originating from a primitive fear of jealous gods. In the fourth century BC, the philosopher Isocrates complained, "One must now apologize for any success in business, as if it were a violation of the moral law, so that today it is worse to prosper than to be a criminal."[21] Lord Bauer, the economist, has dubbed social policies based on pandering to this passion "the economics of resentment," while the sociologist Helmut Schoeck attributed them to the role of envy in human affairs.[22] Blissfully unaware of such works, Singer believes that politically correct claims about "poverty" and "exploitation" articulate perennial truths about "greed" that must be constrained by the benevolent state, aided by selfless intellectuals specializing in the business of human betterment. In short, he preaches the Marxist maxim, "From each according to their ability, to each according to their need," but practices conventional "selfishness."

VI

Viewed in the context of his interest in killing and his admiration for the unsavory medical killer Jack Kevorkian, Singer's avowed interest in saving lives by organ donation is unconvincing, to say the least. The truth is that he is not interested in facilitating organ donation. Instead, he uses this practice to argue that there is no clear line of demarcation between life and death; that the traditional concept of death is an outmoded "fiction [that] is coming apart"; that "the traditional sanctity of life doctrine is increasingly being abandoned by medical practice and the law"; and that we ought to applaud and advance this trend.[23]

Brain-dead persons, Singer declares, "are not persons as I define the term, which is to say, rational and self-aware beings."[24] Singer acknowledges that we use the concept of brain death to justify discontinuing life support and removing organs for transplantation from *live patients,* and use the concept of organismic death for burying or cremating *corpses.* In other words, brain death is the death of a part of the body only. Ordinary language use and social practice refute the inferences Singer draws from the concept of brain death. We do not call brain-dead persons corpses or their bodies "cadavers"; we do not let medical students dissect or undertakers bury their bodies.

Nevertheless, Singer asserts, "With the irreversible loss of consciousness, we have lost everything that we value in our own existence, and everything that gives us reason to hope for the survival of someone we love." Here, Singer transforms his own personal view into an unqualified generalization that is patently false.

Recently, the *Times* of London reported on "legal challenges using the Human Rights Act to defend the right to life . . . Laurence Oates, the Official Solicitor, is expected to argue on behalf of two brain-damaged clients that withdrawing their feeding via tubes breaches their right to life which is guaranteed under the European Convention on Human Rights."[25]

Singer supports his medical-ethical proposals by pretending that the new concept of brain death has displaced, or is about to displace, the old concept of organismic death. This is not true. The two concepts coexist, each serving a very different purpose. Singer refuses to acknowledge that fact, declaring instead, "We cannot go back to the traditional definition of death, for then we would lose the chance to obtain many organs that save people's lives." Obviously, we *could* go back to it, but Singer opposes that option because it would favor the rich over the poor.

If Singer's real goal were to facilitate organ donation, he ought to endorse a free market in organs. Why shouldn't a person be allowed to make provisions for the sale of his organs in case he suffers brain death, much as he is allowed to make provisions for the sale of other property after his demise, the proceeds payable to a beneficiary he names in his will? Why shouldn't he be allowed to sell certain organs, for example, one of his kidneys, while he is still alive, much as he can sell his blood? Singer rejects recognizing that kind of patient autonomy because it conflicts with his "preferences."

VII

Singer's views have been praised by some and condemned by others. His writing is frequently praised as "original and courageous thinking on matters ranging from the treatment of animals to genetic screening."[26] In my judgment, it is neither. His views recast ancient animistic-religious ideas about the "unity of life" as utilitarian bioethics. As for courage, that is a virtue needed by writers who oppose the prevailing liberal-statist style in bioethics, not lead and support it as Singer does.

In what follows, I cite some criticism of Singer that I share. After Singer's controversial appointment to an endowed chair of bioethics at Princeton in 1999, Nat Hentoff, the noted secular civil libertarian, wrote:

> But some of us wondered why Princeton chose this renowned apostle of infanticide and certain forms of euthanasia for so influential an endowed seat at, of all places, the university's Center for Human Values. Professor Singer often claims that his views have been misquoted, so I am quoting directly from his books. From "Practical Ethics": "Human babies are not born self-aware, or capable of grasping that they exist over time. They are not persons." But animals are self-aware, and therefore, "the life of a newborn is of less value than the life of a pig, a dog, or a chimpanzee." Accordingly, from "Should the Baby Live?": "It does not seem wise to add to the burden on limited resources by increasing the number of severely disabled children." Also in that book, Singer and his colleague, Helga Kuhse, suggested that "a period of 28 days after birth might be allowed before an infant is accepted as having the same right to live as others."

Rejecting Singer's philosophical endorsement of killing innocent human beings, Hentoff calls him a "professor of infanticide."[27] Donald De-Marco, professor of philosophy at St. Jerome's College in Toronto, dubs him the "Architect of the Culture of Death."[28] Wesley J. Smith states that "*Rethinking Life and Death* can fairly be called the *Mein Kampf* of the euthanasia movement, in that it drops many of the euphemisms common to pro-euthanasia writing and acknowledges euthanasia for what it is: killing."[29] I agree.

Not the least of Singer's failings as moral philosopher is his ignorance or neglect of writers whose works most effectively refute his views. This is particularly striking in connection with the notion of suffering and the alleged moral imperative to avoid it, which plays such a central role in the calculus of utilitarianism. In his classic *The Liberal Mind* (1963), Kenneth Minogue (1930–) anticipated by some thirty years all that is wrong and wicked about Singer's "practical ethics."[30]

In the index to *Practical Ethics,* Singer lists thirteen separate entries to suffering. He does not mention Minogue's concept of the "suffering situation" and its role in modern liberal politics. Minogue describes his concept of the suffering situation as follows:

> Suffering is a subjective thing, depending on individual susceptibility; politically, it can only be standardized. And it has been standardized, over a long period of time, by an intellectual device which interpreted events in terms of what we may perhaps call a suffering situation. A good example, because morally unambiguous, of a suffering situation would be the condition of child labour in nineteenth-century Britain, or that of slaves in the United States.[31]

One of the suffering situations Singer considers in his book is that experienced by nonhuman animals as a result of humans building a dam: "Thus most of the animals living in the flooded area will die: either they will be drowned, or they will starve. Neither drowning nor starvation are easy ways to die, and the suffering involved in these deaths should, as we have seen, be given *no less weight than we would give to an equivalent amount of suffering experienced by human beings.*"[32] Implicit in Singer's rhetoric is the nonsensical notion that suffering comes in discrete units, like length or weight, and that we possess a metric by which we can compare quantities of suffering experienced by one group with quantities of suffering experienced by another.

Minogue recognized the phoniness of this kind of reasoning intrinsic to utilitarianism: "Liberalism develops from a sensibility which is dissatisfied with the world, not because the world is monotonous, nor because it lacks heroism or beauty, nor because all things are transient, nor for any other of the myriad reasons people find for despair, but because it contains suffering."[33] In this view, progress in civilization is synonymous with reduction in the sum total of suffering, not just of human suffering but of any kind. Accordingly, the crucial distinction is no longer between man and animal, the former having a soul and the ability to reason, and the latter lacking both of these attributes; but rather between living beings that can suffer, such as men and higher animals, and those that cannot, such as plants. "'The question is not,' asks Bentham, 'Can they [animals] *reason?* nor, Can they *talk?* but, Can they *suffer?*'" If we answer yes, the momentous conclusion follows that the "day may come when the rest of the animal creation may acquire these rights which never would have been withholden from them, but by the hand of tyranny."[34]

Minogue also recognized that it is liberalism's misguided concept of, and preoccupation with, suffering situations that has, in part, been responsible for transforming it from its classic, individualistic to its modern collectivistic form:

> Yet even before the end of the nineteenth century, liberal politics began to involve the state in welfare programmes, *converting government from a threat to freedom into an agent of individual happiness.* . . . The suffering of any class of individuals is for liberals a political problem, and politics has been taken as an activity not so much for maximizing happiness as for minimizing suffering. . . . liberalism is good will turned doctrinaire . . . the liberal attitude is entirely secular. It will not countenance theological arguments that suffering in this life is a better passage to heaven than worldly prosperity. . . . Liberals were also a middle group according to their moral interpretation of political life; for while most of society appeared as a complex of groups each struggling for its own interests, *liberals alone were a disinterested force for good, seeking merely to correct what all reasonable men recognized as evils.*[35]

"The suffering of any class of individuals," as Minogue states, "is for liberals a *political* problem, and politics has been taken as an activity not so much for maximizing happiness as for minimizing suffering."[36] The result is a tendency to see suffering as essentially a passive happening, inflicted on "victims" by tyrants, microbes, genes, or "twisted molecules." Suffering is thus robbed of its creative significance; at the same time, persons who suffer are regarded as helpless victims with no means of their own for bearing pain or redressing misfortune: "On the one side we find oppressors, and on the other, a class of victims."[37] This explains why we wage wars not only on literal enemies but also on metaphorical adversaries, such as fear, illness, want, and poverty. In this way the physician is transformed from a healer of the physical ills of individuals into a kind of general who fights a "war" on disease and suffering with a steadily more powerful "armamentarium" of operations, drugs, and mental health services.

The political goals of liberalism and the therapeutic goals of medicine converge on the theme of attending to suffering and trying to abolish it. Both groups consider themselves devoid of partisan passions and self-interests, intent only upon the supra-ethical task of relieving suffering. It is now all too clear how fatally false this view of liberalism is. Yet the idea that therapeutic intention somehow overrules noxious effect, that benevolent motive trumps evil action, is deeply ingrained in the contemporary mind, especially as it relates to the practice of medicine. For example, one writer describes Benjamin Rush as a man who was "laboring to do good even when behaving at his worst" and concludes that "Rush always sought, however violent his therapeutic methods, to be humane."[38]

VIII

My critique of Singer's writings—like my critiques of other collectivistic writings—is based on the Anglo-American philosophy of freedom, with its roots in the works of John Locke, Thomas Jefferson, James Madison, and Lord Acton. Two of the most prominent modern advocates of this philosophy are Ludwig von Mises and Friedrich von Hayek, both self-declared atheists. In this secular-libertarian view, individual liberty and personal responsibility, two sides of the same coin, are the highest ethical-political values. In turn, these values are contingent on the right to property, the sanctity of contract, and the rule of law. Because liberty entails responsibility, it is not conducive to happiness. "If happiness is the end of society," observed Acton, "then liberty is superfluous. It does not make men happy."[39] So much for the utilitarians' glorification of happiness.

In Singer's anticapitalist, collectivist view, the moral legitimacy of private property is suspect and "excess" property exists for the benefit of the anonymous poor, preferably abroad. This contrasts with the classic liberal view, according to which private property exists for the advancement of individual liberty and responsibility and the protection of oneself and one's dependents from future want. We owe the fullest articulation of this ethic to James Madison:

Government is instituted to protect property of every sort; as well as that which lies in the various rights of individuals . . . In its larger and juster meaning, it [property] embraces everything to which a man may attach a value . . . [and includes that] which individuals have in their opinions, their religion, their passions, and their faculties. . . . If the United States mean to obtain and deserve the full praise due to wise and just governments, they will equally respect the rights of property and the property in rights.[40]

Peter Singer wants to cure the disease of being human, a familiar goal that requires a familiar remedy: remaking human nature. The haves should stop spending their money on themselves and their families and spend it, instead, on have-nots who suffer. People should stop killing and eating animals that suffer. Parents and doctors should stop torturing disabled infants and sick people by refusing to kill them and thus causing them more suffering.

It is fitting that Singer is considered the leading ethicist of the therapeutic state.

16

Pharmacracy

The New Despotism

It is doubtful that democracy could survive in a society organized on the
principle of therapy rather than judgment, error rather than sin. If men
are free and equal, they must be judged rather than hospitalized.
—Francis D. Wormuth, *The Origins of Modern
Constitutionalism* (1949)

I

ONE OF THE SYMBOLS of sovereign states is the postage stamp. Traditionally, U.S. stamps have depicted a famous American or an important
historical scene. In 1893, to increase revenues, the U.S. Post Office began to
issue commemorative stamps. The first stamps with a health-related theme—
a stamp depicting children playing and smiling, commemorating the centen-
nial of the American Dental Association—appeared in 1959. In 1999, the
Postal Service unveiled two stamps emblematic of the escalation of America's
wars on diseases. One advertised "Prostate Cancer Awareness: Annual Check-
ups and Tests," the other, "Breast Cancer: Fund the Fight. Find a Cure."[1]

Webster's Third New International Dictionary defines the state as "the
political organization that has supreme civil authority and political power
and serves as the basis of government." Rather than offering definitions
of the state, political scientists prefer to identify its characteristic features,
such as the possession of "organized police powers, defined spatial boundaries, or a formal judiciary . . . [and] a deep and abiding association between the state as a form of social organization and warfare as a political
and economic policy."[2] I regard monopoly of the legitimate use of force as

the quintessential characteristic of the modern state. In this essay, I focus on the use of such force by physicians acting—explicitly or implicitly, wittingly or unwittingly—as agents of the state.

II

The need to justify the use of force seems instinctive. For the child, the parents' power to coerce—by word or deed, intimidation or punishment—appears justified by their superior wisdom, the child's innate lawlessness, and his perception of the socially imposed duty to become domesticated. Thus, the combination of the "natural" authority of superiors, the innate nonconformity of subordinates and their need to learn the rules of the game and adhere to them, and the importance of the welfare of the group (family, society, nation) resting on conformity to social convention form the template for religious, political, and medical justifications of coercive domination.

The result is three familiar ideologies of legitimation: theocracy (God's will); democracy (consent of the governed); and socialism (economic equality, "social justice"). In 1963, I called attention to a novel ideology of legitimation developing in the West, the ideology of pharmacracy animating the therapeutic state and justifying its antilibertarian principles and practices.[3] Since then, I have described and documented the characteristic features of this polity: medical symbols playing the role formerly played by patriotic symbols and the rule of medical discretion and "therapy" replacing the rule of law and punishment.[4]

Undeniably, the state is primarily an apparatus of coercion with a monopoly of the legitimate use of violence. "Government," warned George Washington, "is not reason; it is not eloquence. It is force. Like fire it is a dangerous servant and a fearful master."[5] As the reach of the legitimate influence of this "fearful master" expands, the sphere of personal liberties contracts. What, then, ought to belong to the state, and what to the individual? The history of the West may be viewed in part as the history of the growth of freedom, characterized by a lively debate about where to draw the line between the state's duty to safeguard the interests of the community and its obligation to protect individual liberty. Accustomed to hearing phrases such as "freedom of religion," "freedom of speech," and "the free market," we recognize that each refers to a set of activities free from interference by the coercive apparatus of the state. Should we similarly possess "freedom to be sick," "freedom to make ourselves sick," "freedom to treat ourselves," "freedom to obtain medical care on our own terms," and so forth?

Informed debate about where to draw the line between the welfare of the community and the health of the individual requires that we be clear about the legal distinction between public health and private health. Edward P. Richards and Kathrine C. Rathbun—a law professor and a public health physician, respectively—explain: "Public health is not about making individuals healthy; it is about keeping society healthy by preventing individuals from doing things that endanger others."[6] Hence, preserving and promoting public health often require coercion, whereas preserving and promoting private health require liberty and responsibility. "Persuading people to wear seatbelts, treat their hypertension, eat a healthy diet, and stop smoking," Richards and Rathbun continue, "is personal health protection. Stopping drunk drivers, treating tuberculosis, condemning bad meat, and making people stop smoking where others are exposed to their smoke is public health . . . *Public health should be narrowly defined* in terms of controlling the spread of communicable diseases in society."[7] Instead of confronting the differences and conflicts between public health and private health, politicians, physicians, and laypeople debate slogans, such as the right to health, the patient's bill of rights, patient autonomy, and the wars on drugs, cancer, diabetes, and mental illness.

III

In the nineteenth century, when scientific medicine was in its infancy, disease was defined by pathologists; effective remedies were virtually nonexistent; and the term "treatment" meant medical care sought and paid for by the patient. Today, when scientific medicine is a robust adult, disease is defined by psychiatrists, politicians, and journalists; physicians routinely effect near-miraculous cures; the term "treatment" is regularly used in lieu of the term "coercion"; persons receiving medical treatment are now called "consumers of health services," not patients; and virtually everything called "medical care" is paid for, directly or indirectly, by the state.

The illnesses first conquered by scientific medicine were the infectious diseases. Because the response of the immune system to pathogenic micro-organisms is readily analogized to a nation resisting an invading army, the military or war metaphor has become congenial in thinking about illness and treatment. When we speak about microbes "attacking" the body, antibiotics as magic "bullets," doctors as "fighting" against diseases, and so forth, we use metaphors to convey the idea that the doctor is like the soldier who *protects the homeland from foreign invaders.* However, when we speak about the war on drugs or the war on mental illness, we use metaphors to convey the idea that the state is like a doctor when it uses doctors as soldiers to *protect people from themselves.* In one case, we speak about doctors *helping patients to overcome diseases,* in the other about doctors *preventing citizens from doing what they want to do.*

In the case of infectious diseases—the microbe as alien pathogen threatening the patient's body—the war metaphor helps us understand the mechanism of the disease and justifies the coercive quarantine of contagious persons, animals, or materials. In the case of psychiatric diseases—the war metaphor casting the mental patient in the role of alien pathogen threatening society—the metaphor prevents us from understanding the problem misidentified as a disease: it convinces the patient's family, society, and sometimes the patient himself that the mental patient is (like) a pathogen, justifying the coercive segregation of the subject as "dangerous to himself or others." Failure to understand the abuses of the military metaphor in medicine precludes perceiving medical coercion as a problem.

Viewing the state as primarily an apparatus of coercion with a monopoly of the legitimate use of force does not commit one to denying that the state can do good as well as evil. Moreover, doing evil to some persons often benefits others. The paradigmatic organ of the state is the army, which Robert Heinlein aptly characterized as "a permanent organization for the destruction of life and property."[8] The fact that soldiers are also deployed to rescue people and help guard property after natural disasters does not alter their primary role.

It took centuries of terrible wars before people began to recognize that because the state is par excellence an instrument of violence and because the church ought to be par excellence an instrument of nonviolence, the two should get a divorce or at least a legal separation. By the same token, medicine and the state should also get a divorce. However, Americans do not view the relationship between medicine and the state the same way they view the relationship between church and state. The reason may be that physical illness qua infectious disease, unlike spiritual illness qua "suicidal depression," can directly affect the physical health of the group. That danger has justified certain public health measures as legitimate instruments of state control and coercion. However, this reasoning does not justify state coercion as a morally legitimate instrument for protecting people from themselves. What should be the role of the state with respect to protecting the individual from diseases that do not by themselves pose a threat to others?

Should protecting one's health be the responsibility of individuals, just as it is their responsibility to feed and house themselves and provide for their spiritual health? Should the state assume responsibility for providing "health care" as it used to assume responsibility for providing "religious care"? Should it assume responsibility for protecting individuals from themselves if in the opinion of medical-psychiatric experts they pose a danger to their own health and well-being? In my view, the coercive apparatus of the state ought to be as separate from the professional treatment of medical illness as it is from professional treatment of spiritual illness. Such a separation of medicine and the state is necessary for the protection of our traditional rights to life, liberty, and property.

IV

To understand our present medical-political situation, we must understand the growth of the American state, especially during and since the Roosevelt years. That was when the United States began to become a bureaucratic, regulatory welfare state, a condition brought about by means of the time-honored political tactic of declaring "national emergencies" that required that all of the state's "human resources" be mobilized. "Every collective revolution," warned Herbert Hoover (1874–1964), "rides in on a Trojan horse of 'Emergency.' It was the tactic of Lenin, Hitler, and Mussolini. . . . This technique of creating emergency is the greatest achievement that demagoguery attains."[9] The infamous George Jacques Danton (1759–1794) declared,

"Everything belongs to the fatherland when the fatherland is in danger."[10] Two years later, the fatherland repossessed his head. To the executioner about to guillotine him, he said, "Show my head to the people."[11]

In *Crisis and Leviathan*, Robert Higgs expands on this theme: "Knowing how the government has grown, requires an examination of what, exactly, the government does: the growth of government has resulted not so much from doing more to accomplish traditional governmental functions; rather, it has resulted largely from the government's taking on new functions, activities, and programs—some of them completely novel, others previously the responsibility of the private citizen."[12] Higgs's thesis is that government expansion has been nurtured by a succession of "crises" that the government proceeds to "fix." After a crisis subsides, the new government functions remain, heaping bureaucracies upon bureaucracies. Although Higgs does not include health emergencies among the crises he discusses, they belong on top of the list.

Despite the evidence I have presented, well-respected social analysts maintain that the power and scope of the state are dwindling. In *The Rise and Decline of the State*, Martin van Creveld, a professor of history at Hebrew University in Jerusalem, writes, "The state, which since the middle of the seventeenth century has been the most important and most characteristic of all modern institutions, is in decline."[13] How does Creveld arrive at this conclusion? By emphasizing the increasing popular resistance to the cost of socialist-inspired welfare-state measures, and by ignoring the growing popularity of a medically rationalized therapeutic state. Although Creveld's book runs to 438 pages, he does not mention the war on drugs or the pervasive influence of psychiatric-social controls. Others celebrate the "retreat of the state"—for example, Arthur Seldon, Susan Strange, and Dennis Swann, each of whose book is titled *The Retreat of the State*.[14] I agree with economist Robert J. Samuelson's observation that the government is "getting bigger because, paradoxically, we think it's getting smaller."[15] That curious outcome is just one of the results of the politicization of medicine and of the medicalization of politics.

From 1776 until 1914, when the first antinarcotic legislation was enacted, the federal government played virtually no role in civilian medicine. Medical licensure and the funding and management of state mental hospitals were functions of the state governments. After World War II, the situation changed rapidly and radically: the establishment of the National Institutes of Health, the enactment of Medicare and Medicaid legislation, and the war on drugs soon made medical expenditures the largest component of the national budget, eclipsing defense. The following statistics illustrate the explosive growth of the therapeutic state since the end of World War II and especially since the early 1960s.

In 1950, funding for the National Institute of Mental Health was less than $1 million; ten years later, it was $87 million; by 1992, it reached $1 billion. In 1965, when Medicare and Medicaid were enacted, their cost was $65 billion, rising in 1993 to $939 billion. Between 1969 and 1994, the national mental health budget increased from about $3 billion to $80 billion. Between 1968 and 1983, the number of clinical psychologists tripled, from 12,000 to more than 40,000; the number of clinical social workers grew from 25,000 in 1970 to 80,000 in 1990; and membership in the American Psychological Association grew from fewer than 3,000 in 1970 to more than 120,000 in 1993.[16]

Between 1960 and 1996, the "national health expenditures" share of the gross domestic product (GDP) rose about two and a half times, from 5.1 percent to 13.6 percent. During the same period, the share of "federal government expenditures" on health rose more than six times, from 3.3 percent of the GDP to 20.7 percent. In 1995, total health expenditure, as a percentage of the GDP, was 13.6 percent in the United States, 10.4 percent in Germany, 8.6 percent in Australia, and 6.9 percent in the United Kingdom. Between 1960 and 1998, public expenditure on health care per capita increased more than one hundred times, from $35 to $3,633.

The growth of the state is best illustrated by its cost to the taxpayer, that is, the size of federal budget. The following figures are in nominal dollars. In fiscal 1941, before the United States entered World War II, the budget was $13.6 billion; in 2001, the cost of the war on drugs alone was $19 billion. In 1942, the federal budget more than doubled, to $35.1 billion; and in 1943, it was $78.5 billion. In the next thirty-six years, the budget increased about sixteen times, to $1.65 trillion in 1998. According to James M. Buchanan, professor of economics at George Mason University and 1986 Nobel laureate in economics, "In the seven decades from 1900 to

1970, total government spending in real terms increased forty times over, attaining a share of one-third in national product."[17]

The huge expansion of the government after the 1960s is attributable largely to adding civilian medical care to the functions of the state. This transformation of medicine has utterly distorted the relationship between the private and public realms in general, especially the relationship between private patients and private doctors, private health and public health. What makes the expansion of the therapeutic state especially alarming is the widespread belief that the government is niggardly with respect to health care, especially mental health care, a myth fueled largely by the fact that the number of persons housed in buildings called "state mental hospitals" has decreased since the 1960s. I have documented elsewhere that although it is true that fewer people now reside in state hospitals than did thirty years ago, it is an illusion to think that the scope and power of psychiatry have diminished. The number of persons cared for in one way or another by the mental health system has steadily increased since the end of World War II, as have mental health expenditures.[18] Despite these facts, the author of a "special report" in the *American Bar Association Journal* declares, "No one disputes that government support for the treatment of mental illness has dropped to dangerously low levels."[19]

Let us remember here that the United States is the only country explicitly founded on the principle that, in the inevitable contest between the private and public realms, the scope of the former should be wider than that of the latter. That principle is what made America the "land of the free," especially in the nineteenth century. "There is a balance of power," writes Bruce D. Porter, "between the state and civil society. This internal balance of power demarcates the line between the public and the private—*if a thing is public, it is subject to state authority; if it is private, it is not.*"[20] Pharmacrats want to abolish the private realm altogether. "It is the private sphere that is problematic for public health," declares Dan E. Beauchamp, seemingly not realizing that the *private* sphere is none of the business of *public* health.[21]

It is a truism that people have more liberty in proportion as more aspects of their lives are private. The American people invited the state to take over the management of their health, and now they are surprised that they have less control not only over the health care they receive but also over other aspects of their lives. Nor is that the end of these ostensibly unintended consequences. The more tax monies are spent on health care, the more firmly entrenched becomes the idea in the public mind that caring for people's health requires not individual self-control but political control—that is, control by deception, seduction, and coercion. The state commands vast resources of misinformation (propaganda) and seduction (money and other economic rewards) and has a monopoly of legitimate force (the law and the police).

V

Where we draw a line between health and illness and between the private and the public realms defines and determines a great deal about the kinds of lives we live and have an opportunity to live. The individual's protection or failure to protect his private health may help or harm the community. The measures employed to protect or fail to protect the public health may help or harm the individual. The potential conflict between private health and public health is an integral part of the tension between civil society and the state. In his important paper "Sick Individuals and Sick Populations," epidemiologist Geoffrey Rose notes that "a preventive measure which brings much benefit to the population offers little to each participating individual. This has been the history of public health—immunization, the wearing of seat belts, and now the attempt to change various lifestyle characteristics. Of enormous potential importance to the population as a whole, these measures offer very little—particularly in the short term—to each individual."[22]

Dealing with health care as a public good also raises vexing questions about health insurance, such as: Can we create an insurance system that makes every treatment deemed useful or necessary by a physician available to every member of the community? Can we calculate the cost of health insurance if medical science and technology create, and people clamor for, ever more expensive treatments? If people take good care of their health and live longer, what cost do they impose on those who pay their pensions or other old-age benefits? If the community pays for the treatment of those of its members who fall ill, does it not inevitably acquire a claim on its members to try as hard as they can not to fall ill? Doesn't the community also acquire an interest in identifying and penalizing those who frivolously neglect their health or deliberately make themselves ill? Why don't we subject health care coverage funded by tax monies to a means test? And why don't we model health insurance on private casualty insurance with a substantial deductibility clause—the insured being responsible for his own health care up to, say, 10 percent of taxable income, before becoming eligible for reimbursement? Shouldn't we explore the possibilities of returning to a system in which medical care is available mainly or only to those able and willing to pay for it or insure themselves against certain risks, with care for those who could not pay made available on some other basis?

These are difficult questions that people prefer to avoid. Politicians pander to the public with slogans that promise health care benefits without health care responsibilities, and people like that pandering. However, with the increasing cost of health insurance and the mounting dissatisfaction of both patients and doctors with mandated "insurance" schemes for health care coverage, we ought to confront rather than shirk these questions. The truth is that before the federal government went into the business of health care, poor people received free medical services, often of very good quality, at municipal and teaching hospitals. It is doubtful that they receive better care now, but those who can pay often receive worse care than they did formerly. (By "better" and "worse" I refer here to the human, not the technical, quality of the service.) Moreover, physicians are far less proud of or satisfied with being physicians than they were fifty years ago.

Supporters of pharmacratic politics threaten liberty because they obscure or deny the differences between the kinds of risks posed by a public water supply contaminated with cholera bacilli and the risks posed by a private lifestyle that includes the recreational use of a prohibited psychoactive drug. Individuals *cannot choose* to provide themselves with a safe public water supply, but they *can choose* to protect themselves from the hazards of smoking marijuana. What makes coercive health measures justified is not so much that they protect everyone equally but that they do so by means not available to the individual. By the same token, what makes coercive health measures unjustified is not only that they do not protect everyone equally but that they replace personally assumed self-protection by self-control with legal sanctions difficult or impossible to enforce. The rhetoric of cat-egorizing certain groups—typically children or the residents of neglected neighborhoods—as "at risk" needs to be mentioned here. The term implies that the persons in question lack self-control and therefore need the help of the government to protect them from certain kinds of temptations. Health statists on both the left and the right agree.

Gerald Dworkin, for example, believes, "A man may know the facts [about the dangers of smoking], wish to stop, but not have the requisite willpower. . . . In [such a case] there is no theoretical problem. We are not imposing a good on someone who rejects it. *We are simply using coercion to enable people to carry out their own goals.*"[23] Intellectually, this is nonsense. Politically, it is coercive paternalism. The sole means we have for ascertaining that a man wants to stop smoking more than he wants to enjoy smoking is by observing whether he stops or continues to smoke. Moreover, it is irrespon-sible for moral theorists to ignore that prohibitions of "enjoyments" aimed at protecting people from themselves are not only unenforceable but create black markets and horrifying legal abuses.

The idea that the state has a duty to protect people from themselves is an integral part of the authoritarian, religious-paternalistic outlook on life—now favored by many atheists as well. Once people agree that they have identified the one true God, or Good, it follows that they must guard mem-bers of the group, and nonmembers as well, from the temptation to worship false gods or goods. The post-Enlightenment version of this view arose from a secularization of God and the medicalization of good. Once people agree that they have identified the one true reason, it follows that they must guard against the temptation to worship unreason—that is, madness.

V I

Confronted with the problem of "madness," Enlightenment philosophy was ill prepared to defend the rights of the individual. The modern, secular individual has no more right to be a madman than a medieval individual had a right to be a heretic. When madness appeared in its modern guise, in the seventeenth century, the problem it presented resembled not only the problem of heresy but also the problem of disease, especially of the brain. Madness was perceived to be an "illness of the mind," caused by a hypothesized disease of the brain. This image invited the conflation of risks to the public with risks to the self—hence the view of the insane person as "dangerous to himself or others." For centuries, this verbal formula justified involuntary mental hospitalization. There is a large literature on this subject, to which I have contributed my share, and I shall say no more about it here.

Suffice it to say that the answer to the question of whether a person has a "right to be ill"—physically or mentally—*comes down to whether he is viewed as a private person or as public property:* the former has no obligation to the community to be or stay healthy; the latter does have such an obligation. In proportion as medical care is provided by the state, doctors and patients alike cease to be private persons and forfeit their "rights" against the opposing interests of the state. Declares Alan I. Leshner, head of the National Institute of Drug Abuse: "My belief is that today, in 1998, you [the physician] should be put in jail if you refuse to prescribe S.S.R.I.s [Selective Serotonin Reuptake Inhibitors, a type of so-called antidepressant medication] for depression. I also believe that five years from now you should be put in jail if you don't give crack addicts the medication we're working on now."[24] In plain English, Leshner dreams of *coercing physicians to forcibly drug persons who do not want to be their patients.*

History teaches us that we ought to be on guard against embracing power-hungry professionals as our protectors and guardians. Transforming the United States from a constitutional republic into a therapeutic state has shifted the internal balance of power in favor of the government and against the individual. Ironically, this shift has been accompanied by widespread complaints about a surfeit of autonomy plaguing Americans, by cognoscenti such as Willard Gaylin and Bruce Jennings, authors of *The Perversion of Autonomy: The Proper Uses of Coercion and Constraints in a Liberal Society.*[25] These authors mistake for autonomy what is in fact selfishness engendered by the growth of pharmacratic regulations and the therapeutic state. (I use the term "pharmacratic regulations" to refer to coercive controls exercised by bureaucratic health care regulations and enforced by health care personnel, such as addiction treatment programs, school psychology, and suicide prevention.)

The criminal law tells us that the difference between depriving a person of liberty and depriving him of life is a matter of degree, not kind. The history of religious persecution teaches the same lesson more dramatically. Medical ethicists and psychiatrists ignore this evidence: they embrace medicalized deprivation of liberty, provided it is called "hospitalization," "outpatient commitment," "drug treatment," and so forth. Many, moreover, approve also of medicalized deprivation of life, provided it is called "euthanasia" or "physician-assisted suicide." Once again, we cannot grapple with these problems unless we have clear criteria for the differences between a medical *intervention* and a medical *treatment*. From a scientific point of view, an intervention counts as treatment only if its aim is to remedy a true disease; the identity of the person doing the remedying does not matter: self-medication with an analgesic for pain or with an antihistamine for hay fever counts as treatment. From a legal point of view, an intervention counts as treatment only if it is performed by a physician licensed to practice medicine, with the consent of the subject or his guardian; disease, diagnosis, and medical benefit are irrelevant. Consensual treatment is treatment only if the patient has a true disease, regardless of whether that treatment is effective or does more harm than good. Nonconsensual "treatment" is assault, even if it cures the patient of his disease.

VII

Bedazzled by the myth of mental illness and seduced by psychiatry's usefulness for disposing of unwanted persons, the modern mind recoils from confronting the irreconcilable conflict between the political ideals of a free society and the coercive practices of psychiatry. Let us keep in mind that psychiatry began as a statist enterprise: the insane asylum was a public institution, supported by the state and operated by employees of the state. The main impetus for converting private health into public health came and continues to come from psychiatrists. The history of Nazi Germany as a prototherapeutic state illustrates the truth of that statement.[26]

In 1933, the year Hitler assumed power, a law was passed against "compulsive criminality . . . enabling preventive detention and castration. . . . [for] schizophrenia, manic-depression, [etc.] . . . The medical profession and especially psychiatrists benefited greatly from the drive for sterilization."[27] Reich Health Leader (*Reichgesundheitsführer*) Leonardo Conti (1900–1945) stated, "No one has the right to regard health as a personal private matter, which could be disposed of according to individualistic preference. Therapy has to be administered in the interests of the race and society rather than of the sick individual."[28]

In 1939, medical killing in Germany went into high gear. "Reliable helpers were recruited from the ranks of psychiatrists," who defined lying for the state as a higher form of morality: "Each euthanasia institution had a registry office to issue the false [death] certificates." Modern diagnostic technology was employed as a tool for determining who qualified for therapeutic killing: "In occupied Poland and the Soviet Union, SS X-ray units sought out the tubercular, who were then shot. It is estimated that 100,000 died in this way."[29]

The more power physicians exercised, the more intoxicated with power they became. "The doctor was to be a Führer of the *Volk* to better personal and racial health. . . . Terms like 'euthanasia' and 'the incurable' were a euphemistic medicalized camouflage with connotations of relief of the individual suffering of the terminally ill."[30] Amid the carnage, the Nazis remained obsessed with health: "A plantation for herbal medicines was established at the Dachau concentration camp."

In *The Nazi War on Cancer*, Robert N. Proctor, professor of history at Pennsylvania State University, notes but rejects the similarities between pharmacratic controls in Nazi Germany and in the United States today: "My intention is not to argue that today's anti-tobacco efforts have fascist roots, or that public health measures are in principle totalitarian, as some libertarians seem to want us to believe."[31] Proctor's systematic labeling of Nazi health measures as "fascist" is as misleading as it is politically correct. Hitler was not a fascist, and National Socialism was not a fascist movement. It was a socialist movement wrapped in the flag of nationalism. The terms "fascist" and "fascism" belong to Mussolini and Franco and their movements, neither of which exhibited the kind of interest in eugenics and genocide exhibited by Hitler and the Nazis.

Proctor steers clear of discussing psychiatric practices in Nazi Germany, such as the following typical episode, even though they closely resemble psychiatric practices in the United States today. A father, a retired philologist, complains about the sudden death of his physically healthy schizophrenic son, Hans. He writes to the head of the institution where Hans had been confined, complaining that the explanation for his death was "contrary to the truth" and that "this affair appears to be rather murky." The psychiatrist replies, "The content of your letter . . . forces me to consider psychiatric measures against you. . . . should you continue to harass us with further communications, I shall be forced to have you examined by a public health physician."[32] As Proctor himself shows, it was principally psychiatry that provided the "scientific" justification and personnel for medical mass murder in Nazi Germany. Nevertheless, he declares, "I should reassure the reader that I have no desire to efface the brute and simple facts—the complicity in crime or the sinister stupidities of Nazi ideology."[33] Calling Nazi ideology "stupid" is like calling a distasteful religious belief "stupid." It is a narrow-minded refusal to understand the Other's ideology on its own terms, as if understanding it were tantamount to approving it. The truth is that the Nazi health ideology closely resembles the present American health ideology. Each rests on the same premise—that individuals are incompetent to protect themselves from themselves and need the protection of the paternalistic state, thus turning private health into public health. Proctor is too eager to efface the method in the madness of the Nazis' *furor therapeuticus politicus,* perhaps because it is so alarmingly relevant to our version of it.

"Nazism itself," he writes, "I will be treating as . . . a vast hygienic experiment designed to bring about an exclusionist sanitary utopia. That sanitary utopia was a vision not unconnected with fascism's more familiar genocidal aspects."[34] It was fanatical medical puritanism, not fascism, that motivated the Nazis to wage therapeutic wars against cancer, homosexuals, Gypsies, and Jews. This is a crucial point. Once we begin to worship health as an all-pervasive good—a moral value that trumps all others, especially liberty—we sanctify it as a kind of secular holiness.

With respect to the relationship between health and the state, Hitler's goal was the same as Plato's and the modern public health zealots'—namely, abolishing the boundary between private and public health. Here are some striking examples, all of which Proctor misleadingly interprets as manifestations of "fascism": "Your body belongs to the nation! Your body belongs to the Führer! You have the duty to be healthy! Food is not a private matter! (National Socialist slogans.) . . . We have the duty, if necessary, to die for the Fatherland; why should we not also have the duty to be healthy? Has the Führer not explicitly demanded this? . . . Nicotine damages not just the individual but the population as a whole."[35]

Hitler and his entourage were health fanatics obsessed with cleanliness and with killing "bugs," the latter category including unwanted people, especially mental patients. Hitler neither drank nor smoked and was a vegetarian. Preoccupied with the fear of illness and the welfare of animals, he could not "tolerate the idea of animals' being killed for human consumption."[36] After Hitler became chancellor, Reichsmarshall Hermann Göring announced an end to the "unbearable torture and suffering in animal experiments." The medical mass murder of mental patients went hand in hand with the prohibition of vivisection, which was declared a capital offense. The fact that the Nazi public health ethic demanded not only respect for the health of the greatest numbers (of Aryans) but also for the health of animals (except "bugs") illustrates the connections between the love of pharmacracy and animal rights, on one hand, and the loathing of human rights and the lives of imperfect persons, on the other hand, as the writings of bioethicist Peter Singer illustrate.[37]

Instead of viewing the Nazi experience with medicalized politics as a cautionary tale illuminating the dangers lurking in the alliance between medicine and the state, Proctor uses it to speculate about what the Nazi war on cancer "tells us about the nature of fascism." He arrives at the comforting conclusion that "the Nazi analogy is pretty marginal to contemporary discussions about euthanasia" and criticizes "pro-tobacco activists"—as if opposing antitobacco legislation made one automatically a "pro-tobacco activist"—who "play the Nazi card."[38] Our future liberty, and health as well, may depend on whether we dismiss the analogy between pharmacracy in Nazi Germany and pharmacracy in contemporary America as "pretty marginal," as Proctor believes we should, or whether, as I suggest, we view it as of the utmost relevance and treat it accordingly.

When health is equated with freedom, liberty as a political concept vanishes. We understand and accept the person who prefers security over liberty, but we do not understand or accept the person who prefers disease over health, death over life.

VIII

The collectivization of American medicine, like the collectivization of much else in America, began during the presidency of Franklin D. Roosevelt. In 1940, in a speech delivered at the dedication of the newly established National Institutes of Health, Roosevelt declared, "The defense this nation seeks involves a great deal more than building airplanes, ships, guns, and bombs. We cannot be a strong nation unless we are a healthy nation."[39] With equal justification, Roosevelt might have said, "We cannot be a strong nation unless we are a prosperous nation."

We have become a prosperous nation by separating the economy and the state, not by making the state the source of employment, as have the communists, with the disastrous results now known to all. We can become a healthy nation only by separating medicine and the state, not by making the state the source of health care, as have the communists, with similarly disastrous results.

Long before the reign of modern totalitarianisms, English economist and statesman Richard Cobden (1804–1865) warned, "They who propose to influence by force the traffic of the world, forget that affairs of trade, like matters of conscience, change their very nature if touched by the hand of violence; for as faith, if forced, would no longer be religion, but hypocrisy, so commerce becomes robbery if coerced by warlike armaments."[40] The same principle applies to medicine. As "affairs of trade. . . . change their very nature if touched by the hand of violence," so affairs of medicine also change their very nature if touched by the hand of violence and, if forced, cease to be forms of treatment and become, instead, forms of tyranny.

Americans' love affair with pharmacracy now transcends traditional distinctions between left and right, liberal and conservative, Democrat and Republican. Physicians, who ought to know better but for the most part don't, are perhaps the most naive and at the same time the most zealous advocates of medical interventions for all manner of human problems. Writing in the *Journal of the American Medical Association,* two physicians plead for a "comprehensive public health surveillance of firearm injuries." Why? Because "firearm injuries are a leading cause of death and disability in the United States."[41] We are building a society based on the false premise that if X is a "leading cause" of death, then X is a disease and a public health problem whose prevention and treatment justify massive infringements on personal freedom.

The leading cause of death is being alive. The therapeutic state swallows all life on the seemingly rational ground that nothing falls outside the province of health and medicine, just as the theological state had swallowed up everything human on the ground that nothing falls outside the province of God and religion. Lest it seem that I exaggerate the parallels between these two types of total states and the religious nature of the therapeutic state, consider Vice President Al Gore's by no means atypical remarks, offered in an address at Emory University on June 1, 2000. Pledging to wage the war on cancer with renewed vigor, he declared, "Within ten years, no one in America should have to die from colon cancer, breast cancer, or prostate cancer. . . . The power to fight cancer comes from the heart and from the human spirit. But most of all, it comes from being able to imagine a day when you are cancer-free." His Web site carried his message under the banner headline, "Gore Sets Goal for a Cancer-Free America."[42] Thus do Christian Science and the wars on diseases blend into political vapidity and pharmacratic tyranny.

America's drift toward pharmacracy has not escaped the attention of some perceptive social commentators. "Our politicians," observes Andrew Ferguson, "are transcending politics. . . . How is it . . . that politicians who for years promised to keep government out of our bedrooms now see fit to invite their way into our souls? They have cast themselves as empaths; soul-fixing is their job. . . . Their bet is that America today wants a Therapist in Chief."[43]

Indeed, Americans want a therapist-in-chief who is both physician and priest, an authority that will protect them from having to assume responsibility not only for their own health care but also for their behaviors that make them ill, literally or figuratively. Pandering to this passion, politicians assure people that they have a "right to health" and that their maladies are "no-fault diseases"; promise them a "patient's bill of rights" and an America "free of cancer" and "free of drugs"; and stupefy them with an inexhaustible torrent of mind-altering prescription drugs and mind-numbing anti-disease and anti-drug propaganda—as if anyone could be *for* illness or drug abuse.

Formerly, people rushed to embrace totalitarian states. Now they rush to embrace the therapeutic state. By the time they discover that the therapeutic state is about tyranny, not therapy, it will be too late.

NOTES

SELECTED BIBLIOGRAPHY

INDEX

Notes

PREFACE

1. Daniel L. Dreisbach, "Origins and Dangers of the 'Wall of Separation' Between Church and State," *Imprimis,* October 2006, http://www.hillsdale.edu/imprimis/2006/10/, emphasis added (accessed April 15, 2007).

INTRODUCTION

1. Linda Landesman, "Banning Trans Fats," *New York Times,* October 7, 2006, http://www.nytimes.com/2006/10/07/opinion/l07fat.html.

2. Thomas Szasz, *The Myth of Mental Illness: Foundations of a Theory of Personal Conduct* [1961], rev. ed. (New York: HarperCollins, 1974).

3. E. Kinetz, "Is Hysteria Real? Brain Images Say Yes," *New York Times,* September 26, 2006.

4. J. Windolf, "A Nation of Nuts," *Wall Street Journal,* October 22, 1997. Reprinted at http://www.brianwilson.net/pages/nuts.html (accessed April 15, 2007).

5. Anton Chekhov, "Ward No. 6" [1892], in Thomas Szasz, ed., *The Age of Madness: The History of Involuntary Mental Hospitalization Presented in Selected Texts* (Garden City, N.Y.: Doubleday, 1973), 89–126, 100–101.

6. Jules Romains, *Knock (Knock, ou le triomphe de médecine),* trans. James B. Gidney (1923; Great Neck, N.Y.: Barron Educational Series, 1962), 12, 35.

7. Robert Jay Lifton, *The Nazi Doctors: Medical Killing and the Psychology of Genocide,* http://www.holocaust-history.org/lifton/contents.shtml (accessed April 15, 2007).

8. Charles E. Rosenberg, "Contested Boundaries: Psychiatry, Disease, and Diagnosis," *Perspectives in Biology and Medicine* 49 (Summer 2006): 407–24.

9. Gilbert Ryle, *The Concept of Mind* (London: Hutchinson's University Library, 1949).

10. Szasz, *The Myth of Mental Illness.*

11. Emil Kraepelin, *Lectures on Clinical Psychiatry* [1901] (New York: Hafner, 1968), 1; *Einführung in die psychiatrische Klinik* (Leipzig: Johann Ambrosius Barth, 1901), 1, emphasis added.

12. Ernst von Feuchtersleben, *Medical Psychology* (1845), in Daniel Schreber, *Memoirs of My Nervous Illness* [1903], trans. Ida Macalpine and Richard Hunter (London: William Dawson and Sons, 1955), 412.

13. See Anna Freud, *Normality and Pathology in Childhood: Assessments of Development* (New York: International Universities Press, 1965), 120.

14. Sigmund Freud, *The Psychopathology of Everyday Life* (1901), in *The Standard Edition of the Complete Psychological Works of Sigmund Freud,* trans. James Strachey (London: Hogarth Press, 1953–74), vol. 6. Cited hereafter as *SE.*

15. Sigmund Freud, *The Question of Lay Analysis* (1927), *SE,* 20:229.

16. Sigmund Freud, "On the History of the Psychoanalytic Movement" (1914), *SE,* 14:66.

17. Sigmund Freud, *New Introductory Lectures on Psychoanalysis* (1932–36), *SE,* 22:153.

18. Sigmund Freud, *An Autobiographical Study* (1924), *SE,* 20:25.

19. Freud, *New Introductory Lectures,* 152.

20. Ibid., 252.

21. Ibid., 230.

22. Ibid., 184.

23. Sigmund Freud, *An Outline of Psychoanalysis* (1938–1940), *SE,* 23:77.

24. Freud, *The Psychopathology of Everyday Life,* 254.

25. Freud, *The Psychopathology of Everyday Life.*

26. Richard von Krafft-Ebing, *Psychopathia Sexualis, with Special Reference to the Antipathic Sexual Instinct: A Medico-Forensic Study* [1886, 1906]. Authorized English adaptation of the twelfth German edition by F. J. Rebman, rev. ed. (Brooklyn, NY: Physicians and Surgeons Book Company, 1931), vi, vii, emphasis added.

27. Ibid., 52–54.

28. Thomas Szasz, *Sex by Prescription: The Startling Truth about Today's Sex Therapy* [1980] (Syracuse: Syracuse University Press, 1990).

29. William Masters and Virginia Johnson, *Human Sexual Inadequacy* (Boston: Little, Brown, 1970), 150.

30. Thomas Szasz, *Coercion as Cure: A Critical History of Psychiatry* (New Brunswick, NJ: Transaction, 2007).

31. Johnson Institute, "Future Bright for Recovery, Experts Say: Johnson Institute National Forum Draws Leading Innovators in Field," November 24, 2004, http://johnson institute.org/Events/Proceedings.aspx?id=88 (accessed April 15, 2007).

32. DepressionIsReal.org, http://www.depressionisreal.org/ (accessed April 15, 2007).

33. http://www.dbsalliance.org/dir.htm (accessed April 15, 2007).

34. The Depression Is Real Coalition, "Education Campaign to Counter Misconceptions about Depression," http://www.nami.org/Template.cfm?Section=Press_September_ 2006&Template=/ContentManagement/ContentDisplay.cfm&ContentID=38422, emphasis added (accessed April 15, 2007).

35. National Mental Health Association, "Finding Hope & Help: College Student and Depression Pilot Initiative," http://www.nmha.org/camh/college/index.cfm, emphasis added (accessed April 15, 2007).

36. Abraham Lincoln, "Fragment: On Slavery," October 1, 1858, http://teaching americanhistory.org/library/index.asp?document=1058 (accessed April 15, 2007).

37. Quoted in Erik J. Engstrom, *Clinical Psychiatry in Imperial Germany: A History of Psychiatric Practice* (Ithaca, N.Y.: Cornell University Press, 2003), 251.

I. MENTAL ILLNESS: A METAPHORICAL DISEASE

1. Thomas Szasz, *The Myth of Mental Illness: Foundations of a Theory of Personal Conduct* (New York: Hoeber-Harper, 1961; London: Secker & Warburg, 1962; London: Paladin, 1972).

2. Sigmund Freud, "Some Points for a Comparative Study of Organic and Hysterical Paralyses" (1893), in *The Standard Edition of the Complete Psychological Works of Sigmund Freud*, trans. James Strachey (London: Hogarth Press, 1953–74), 1:155–72, 162. Hereafter cited as *SE*.

3. Ibid., 169.

4. Joseph Breuer and Sigmund Freud, "On the Psychical Mechanism of Hysterical Phenomena: Preliminary Communication" (1893), in *SE*, 2:1–17, 7.

5. Sigmund Freud, "Some General Remarks on Hysterical Attacks," *SE*, 9:227–34; 229.

6. Thomas Szasz, *The Manufacture of Madness: A Comparative Study of the Inquisition and the Mental Health Movement* (New York: Harper & Row, 1970).

7. *The Guardian*, May 20, May 22, 1972.

8. *Sunday Telegraph*, June 11, 1972.

9. *Sunday Times*, July 2, 1972; *New Statesman*, July 7 and 8, 1972.

2. MENTAL ILLNESS: THE NEW PHLOGISTON

1. Arthur Donovan, *Antoine Lavoisier: Science, Administration, and Revolution* (Oxford: Blackwell, 1993).

2. Joseph Priestley, *Considerations on the Doctrine of Phlogiston and the Decomposition of Water* (Philadelphia: Thomas Dobson, 1796), http://www.web.lemoyne.edu/~giunta/priest ley.html (accessed April 15, 2007).

3. Henry Maudsley quoted in E. H. Reynolds and M. R. Trimble, eds., *Epilepsy and Psychiatry* (London: Churchill Livingstone, 1981), 4.

4. Michael S. Moore, "Some Myths about 'Mental Illness,'" *Archives of General Psychiatry* 32 (1975): 1483–97.

5. Thomas Szasz, "'Audible Thoughts' and 'Speech Defect' in Schizophrenia: A Note on Reading and Translating Bleuler," *British Journal of Psychiatry* 168 (1996): 533–35.

6. Thomas Szasz, *The Meaning of Mind: Language, Morality, and Neuroscience* [1996] (Syracuse: Syracuse University Press, 2002), 124–29.

7. George Hoyer, "On the Justification for Civil Commitment," *Acta Psychiatrica Scandinavica* 101 (2000): 65–71.

8. George J. Alexander and Alan W. Scheflin, *Law and Mental Disorder* (Durham, N.C.: Carolina Academic Press, 1998).

9. R. Wilkinson, "Word-Choosing: Sources of a Modern Obsession," *Encounter* (May 1982): 80–87.

4. DIAGNOSIS: FROM DESCRIPTION TO PRESCRIPTION

1. Alvan R. Feinstein, "ICD, POR, and DRG: Unsolved Scientific Problems in the Nosology of Clinical Medicine," *Archives of Internal Medicine* 148 (1988): 2269–74, emphasis added.

2. Ganesh G. Gupta, "Diagnosis-Related Groups: A Twentieth-Century Nosology," *Pharos* 53 (1990): 12–17.

3. Paul E. Greenberg et al., "The Economic Burden of Depression in 1990," *Journal of Clinical Psychiatry* 54 (1993): 405–17.

4. Tipper Gore, "The High Social Cost of Mental Illness," *Wall Street Journal,* January 12, 1994, p. All.

5. Jose M. Santiago, "The Costs of Treating Depression," *Journal of Clinical Psychiatry* 54 (1993): 425–26.

6. Henry Blissenbach quoted in Milton Freudenheim, "The Drug Makers Are Listening to Prozac," *New York Times,* January 9, 1994, p. E7.

7. I have consulted the following texts, none of which lists depression or schizophrenia in its index or presents them as diseases: John M. Kissane, ed., *Anderson's Pathology,* 9th ed. (Philadelphia: Mosby, 1990); Ramzi S. Cotran, Vinay Kumar, and Stanley L. Robbins, *Robbins Pathologic Basis of Disease,* 4th ed. (Philadelphia: Saunders, 1989); R. A. Crawson et al., *Pathology: The Mechanism of Disease,* 2nd ed. (Philadelphia: Mosby, 1989); Emanuel Rubin and John L. Farber, eds., *Pathology* (Philadelphia: Lippincott, 1988).

8. Tipper Gore, "The High Social Cost of Mental Illness."

9. D. Cauchon,"Attack on the Deadheads Is No Hallucination: Band's Followers Handed Stiff LSD Sentences," *USA Today,* December 17, 1992, p. A6.

10. M. W. Miller,"FDA Clears J & J Schizophrenia Drug," *Wall Street Journal,* January 12, 1994.

11. Ibid.

12. Ibid.

5. DIAGNOSES ARE NOT DISEASES

1. American Psychiatric Association, *Diagnostic and Statistical Manual of Mental Disorders of the American Psychiatric Association* (*DSM-III*), 3rd ed. (Washington, D.C.: American Psychiatric Association, 1980).

2. American Psychiatric Association, *Diagnostic and Statistical Manual of Mental Disorders of the American Psychiatric Association* (*DSM-III-R*), 3rd rev. ed. (Washington, D.C.: American Psychiatric Association, 1987), xvii.

3. American Psychiatric Association, *DSM-IV Options Book: Work in Progress* (Washington, D.C.: American Psychiatric Association, 1991).

4. Thomas Szasz, *The Myth of Mental Illness* [1961], rev. ed. (New York: Harper and Row, 1974).

5. Editorial, "British Psychiatry at 150," *Lancet* 338 (September 28, 1991): 785–86, 785.

6. Michael Polanyi, "Life's Irreducible Structures" [1968], in Polanyi, *Knowing and Being: Essays by Michael Polanyi,* ed. Marjorie Grene (Chicago: University of Chicago Press, 1969), 238.

7. Ibid.

8. Milton Freudenheim, "New Law to Bring Wider Job Rights for Mentally Ill," *New York Times,* September 23, 1991, pp. A1, D4.

9. Will Rogers, "The Congressional Record" [1935], in *A Will Rogers Treasury: Reflections and Observations,* ed. Bryan B. and Frances N. Sterling (New York: Bonanza Books, 1982), 256.

10. Freudenheim, "New Law to Bring Wider Job Rights for Mentally Ill."

11. Milton Freudenheim, "At Work, a New Deal for the Mentally Ill," *Wall Street Journal,* September 24, 1991.

12. M. J. Goldman,"Kleptomania: Making Sense out of Nonsense," *American Journal of Psychiatry* 148 (August 1991): 986–96.

13. Ibid., 986, emphasis added.

14. Thomas Szasz, *Insanity: The Idea and Its Consequences* (New York: Wiley, 1987).

15. C. Miller, "Course Offers Cure for Shoplifting," *Syracuse Herald-Journal,* October 17, 1991, p. B1.

16. Ibid., emphasis added.

17. L. Bien, "Addicted Shoppers Attempt to Buy Happiness," *Syracuse Herald-Journal,* October 23, 1991, pp. C1, C3, C1.

18. Ibid., p. C3.

19. *DSM-III-R,* 255.

20. Ibid., 269.

21. Ibid., 283.

22. Ibid., 293.

23. Ibid., 316.

24. Richard Karel, "Controversy Follows DWI Acquittal Based on Premenstrual Syndrome Defense," *Psychiatric News* 26 (September 6, 1991): 16–18.

25. Ibid., 18.

26. Ibid., 18.

27. Szasz, *Insanity,* especially 9–98.

6. THE EXISTENTIAL IDENTITY THIEF

1. Bertrand Russell, *A History of Western Philosophy: And Its Connection with Political and Social Circumstances from the Earliest Times to the Present Day* (New York: Simon and Schuster, 1945), 673.

2. Bertrand Russell, *Sceptical Essays* (London: Allen & Unwin, 1928), 1.

3. Clive S. Lewis, *Mere Christianity* (New York: Macmillan, 1952), 40–41.

7. DEFINING DISEASE

1. Thomas Szasz, *Pharmacracy: Medicine and Politics in America* (2001; Syracuse: Syracuse University Press, 2003).

2. Thomas Szasz, *The Therapeutic State: Psychiatry in the Mirror of Current Events* (Buffalo: Prometheus Books, 1984).

3. Thomas Szasz, *The Manufacture of Madness: A Comparative Study of the Inquisition and the Mental Health Movement* (1970; Syracuse: Syracuse University Press, 1997).

4. Thomas Szasz, *The Untamed Tongue: A Dissenting Dictionary* (LaSalle, Ill.: Open Court, 1990), 160.

5. L. B. Yeager, "From Gold to the ECU: The International Monetary System in Retrospect," *Independent Review* 1 (Spring 1996): 75–99.

6. John M. Keynes, *The Economic Consequences of the Peace* [1920]. Introduction by Robert Lekachman (New York: Penguin, 1970), 236.

7. Roy Porter, *Flesh in the Age of Reason: The Modern Foundations of Body and Soul* (New York: Norton, 2004), 308.

8. "Herman Boerhaave," http://www.whonamedit.com/doctor.cfm.2404.html (accessed April 15, 2007).

9. Science Week, "Cognitive Science: From Brain to Mind. 2004," http://scienceweek.com/2004/sa040903-4.htm (accessed April 15, 2007).

10. D. Dennett, *Consciousness Explained* (Boston: Little, Brown, 1991), 31.

11. Alan J. Hobson, *The Chemistry of Conscious States: How the Brain Changes Its Mind* (Boston: Little, Brown, 1994), 6–7.

12. Christian De Duve, *Life Evolving: Molecules, Mind, and Meaning* (New York: Oxford University Press, 2002), 208.

13. Ibid., 200.

14. Ibid., emphasis added.

15. Ibid., 209.

16. Samuel H. Barondes, "The Biological Approach to Psychiatry: History and Prospects," *Journal of Neuroscience* 10 (June 1990): 1707–10; 1709, emphasis added.

17. Benjamin Rush, *Medical Inquiries and Observations Upon the Diseases of the Mind* (1812; New York: Macmillan-Hafner Press, 1962), 350.

18. Richard von Krafft-Ebing, *Psychopathia Sexualis, with Special Reference to the Antipathic Sexual Instinct: A Medico-Forensic Study,* authorized English adaptation of the twelfth German edition by F. J. Rebman, rev. ed. (1886; Brooklyn, N.Y.: Physicians and Surgeons Book Company, 1931).

19. Sigmund Freud, *The Standard Edition of the Complete Psychological Works of Sigmund Freud,* trans. James Strachey (London: Hogarth Press, 1953–74), 24 vols.

20. "Is Extreme Racism a Mental Illness?" *New Crisis* (January–February 2000): 23–25.

21. Frank Tallis quoted in J. Waters, "Love and Madness," *Washington Times,* February 14, 2005.

22. Richard Dobson and S.-K. Templeton, "Love's Not Only Blind but Mad, Say Scientists," *Sunday Times* (London), February 13, 2005.

23. Germund Hesslow, "Do We Need a Concept of Disease?" *Theoretical Medicine* 14 (1993): 1–14, 3, emphasis added.

8. THE ORIGIN OF PSYCHIATRY: COERCION AS CURE

1. See generally William L. Parry-Jones, *The Trade in Lunacy: A Study of Private Madhouses in England in the Eighteenth and Nineteenth Centuries* (London: Routledge & Kegan Paul, 1976).

2. Thomas Szasz, *Law, Liberty, and Psychiatry* [1963] (Syracuse: Syracuse University Press, 1989).

3. Richard Neugebauer, "Diagnosis, Guardianship, and Residential Care of the Mentally Ill in Medieval and Early Modern England," *American Journal of Psychiatry* 111 (December 1989): 1580–84, 1580.

4. Ibid., 1582.

5. Thomas Szasz, *Insanity: The Idea and Its Consequences* (1987; Syracuse: Syracuse University Press, 1997).

6. See M. Orrell, B. Sahakian, and K. Bergmann, "Self-Neglect and Frontal Lobe Dysfunction," *British Journal of Psychiatry* 155 (January 1989): 101–5; and P. Vostanis and C. Dean, "Self-Neglect in Adult Life," *British Journal of Psychiatry* 161 (August 1992): 265–67.

7. Michel Foucault, *Madness and Civilization: A History of Insanity in the Age of Reason* [1961] (New York: Pantheon, 1965).

8. Roy Porter, *Mind-Forg'd Manacles: A History of Madness from the Restoration to the Regency* (London: Athlone Press, 1987), 8–9.

9. Parry-Jones, *The Trade in Lunacy,* 241.

10. Ibid.

11. Roy Porter, *Mind-forg'd Manacles,* 88.

12. Ibid.

13. Richard Hunter and Ida Macalpine, *Three Hundred Years of Psychiatry, 1533–1860: A History Presented in Selected English Texts* (London: Oxford University Press, 1963), 196.

14. George Cheyne, *The English Malady, Or, a Treatise of Nervous Diseases of All Kinds, as Spleen, Vapours, Lowness of Spirits, Hypochondriacal and Hysterical Distempers, etc.* (London: Strahan & Leake, 1733).

15. Ibid., 1.

16. Ibid., 111.

17. "Jerusalem Syndrome," http://en.wikipedia.org/wiki/Jerusalem_syndrome; "Stockholm Syndrome," http://en.wikipedia.org/wiki/Stockholm_syndrome; "'Paris Syndrome' Leaves Japanese Tourists in Shock," http://www.msnbc.msn.com/id/15391010/ (accessed April 15, 2007).

18. See, for example, Nellie Bly (Elizabeth Cochrane), *Ten Days in a Madhouse, or Nellie Bly's Experience on Blackwell's Island. Feigning Insanity in Order to Reveal Asylum Horrors* (New York: Norman L. Munroe, 1887).

19. Daniel Defoe, *Augusta Triumphans* (1728), in Hunter and Macalpine, *Three Hundred Years of Psychiatry,* 266–67.

20. Thomas Szasz, *Cruel Compassion: The Psychiatric Control of Society's Unwanted* [1994] (Syracuse: Syracuse University Press, 1998).

21. Michael DePorte, *Nightmares and Hobbyhorses: Swift, Sterne, and Augustan Ideas of Madness* (San Marino, Calif.: Huntington Library, 1974), 56.

22. Jonathan Swift, *A Tale of a Tub* [1704], in *Jonathan Swift,* ed. Angus Ross and David Woolley (New York: Oxford University Press, 1984), 147–48.

23. Thomas Hobbes, *Leviathan* [1651], ed. Michael Oakeshott (New York: Macmillan/ Collier, 1962), 62.

24. Swift, *A Tale of a Tub,* in *Jonathan Swift,* ed. Ross and Woolley, 141.

25. Irwin Ehrenpreis, *Swift: The Man, His Works, and the Age* (Cambridge: Harvard University Press, 1983), 3:580.

26. E. G. O'Donoghue, *The Story of Bethlehem Hospital, From Its Foundation in 1247* (New York: Dutton, 1915), 249.

27. Ibid., 250.

28. Jonathan Swift, "Verses on the Death of Dr. Swift," in *Jonathan Swift,* ed. Ross and Woolley, 530.

29. E. C. Mossner, "Swift, Jonathan (1667–1745)," in *The Encyclopedia of Philosophy,* ed. Paul Edwards (New York: Macmillan and Free Press, 1967), 8:52.

30. Swift, "Verses on the Death of Dr. Swift," in *Jonathan Swift,* ed. Ross and Woolley, 516.

9. HYSTERIA AS LANGUAGE

1. Joseph Breuer and Sigmund Freud, *Studies on Hysteria* (1893–1905), in *The Standard Edition of the Complete Psychological Works of Sigmund Freud,* ed. James Strachey (London: Hogarth Press, 1953–74), 1:135–36.

2. Ibid., 166.

3. Joseph Rogues De Fursac, *Manual of Psychiatry and Mental Hygiene* (1903), 7th ed. (New York: Wiley, 1938), 317.

10. ROUTINE NEONATAL CIRCUMCISION: A MEDICAL RITUAL

1. Genesis 17:9.

2. 1 Samuel 18:25.

3. Abraham Cohen, *Everyman's Talmud* (New York: Schocken, 1975), 381.

4. Thomas Szasz, *Insanity: The Idea and Its Consequences* [1987] (Syracuse: Syracuse University Press, 1997).

5. Gerald Weiss, "Ritual Circumcision," *Clinical Pediatrics* 1 (October 1962): 65–72.

6. Peter C. Remondino, *History of Circumcision: From the Earliest Times to the Present* (Philadelphia: F. A. Davis, 1891. Reprint; New York: AMS Press, 1974), 147, 157.

7. Moses Maimonides, *The Guide for the Perplexed* (New York: Dover, 1956), 378.

8. Karen E. Paige and Jeffrey M. Paige, *The Politics of Reproductive Ritual* (Berkeley: University of California Press, 1981), 263–67.

9. A. Money, *Treatment of Disease in Children* (Philadelphia: Blakiston, 1887), 421.

10. Thomas Szasz, *The Manufacture of Madness: A Comparative Study of the Inquisition and the Mental Health Movement* [1970] (Syracuse: Syracuse University Press, 1997), 180–206.

11. Edward Wallerstein, *Circumcision: An American Health Fallacy* (New York: Springer, 1980).

12. Edward Wallerstein, "Circumcision: The Uniquely American Medical Enigma," *Urologic Clinics of North America* 12 (February 1985): 123–32, 123.

13. Aaron J. Fink, "Newborn Circumcision: A Long-Term Strategy for AIDS Prevention," *Journal of the Royal Society of Medicine* 83 (October 1990): 673.

14. David M. Feldman, *Birth Control in Jewish Law: Marital Relations, Contraception, and Abortion as Set Forth in the Classical Texts of Jewish Law* (New York: New York University Press, 1968), 114.

15. Louis M. Epstein, *Sex Laws and Customs in Judaism* (New York: Ktav Publishing House, 1967), 137.

16. Szasz, *The Manufacture of Madness,* 182 ff.

17. E. J. Schoen, "Are We Becoming a Two-Class Society Based on Neonatal Circumcision?" (Letter), *Pediatrics* 86 (December 1990): 1005–6.

18. Jules Romains, *Knock* (*Knock, ou le triomphe de médecine*), trans. James B. Gidney (1923; Great Neck, N.Y.: Barron Educational Series, 1962), 35.

19. E. J. Schoen, "The Status of Circumcision of Newborns," *New England Journal of Medicine* 322 (May 3, 1990): 1308–12, 1308.

20. "Minerva," *British Medical Journal* 307 (October 30, 1993): 1154. See also N. W. Williams and L. Kapila, "Complications of Circumcision," *British Journal of Surgery* 80 (October 1993): 1231–36.

21. "Female Genital Cutting," Wikipedia, http://en.wikipedia.org/wiki/Female_circumcision (accessed April 15, 2007).

22. Shannon Brownlee et al., "In the Name of Ritual: An Unprecedented Legal Case Focuses on Genital Politics," *U.S. News & World Report,* February 7, 1994, pp. 56–58; and M. H. Merwine, "How Africa Understands Female Circumcision," *New York Times,* November 24, 1993, p. A24.

23. S. L. Olamijulu, "Female Child Circumcision in Ilesha, Nigeria," *Clinical Pediatrics* 22 (August 1983): 580–81.

24. Editorial, "A Ritual Operation," *British Medical Journal* 1458 (December 24, 1949): 1458.

25. William F. Gee and Julian S. Ansell, "Neonatal Circumcision: A Ten-Year Overview," *Pediatrics* 58 (December 1976): 824–27.

26. Task Force on Circumcision, "Report of the Task Force on Circumcision," *Pediatrics* 84 (August 1989): 388–91, 388.

27. Edgar J. Schoen, "The Relationship Between Circumcision and Cancer of the Penis," *CA: A Cancer Journal for Clinicians* 41 (September–October 1991): 306–9.

28. Thomas E. Wiswell and W. E. Hachey, "Urinary Tract Infections and the Uncircumcised State: An Update," *Clinical Pediatrics* 32 (1993): 130–34.

29. Ingela Bollgren and Jan Winberg, "Reply to 'Is It Time for Europe to Reconsider Newborn Circumcision?'" *Acta Paediatrica Scandinavica* 80 (1991): 573–80.

30. Ronald L. Poland, "The Question of Routine Neonatal Circumcision," *New England Journal of Medicine* 322 (May 3, 1990): 1312–15, 1315, emphasis added.

31. American Medical Association, *Medicolegal Forms with Legal Analysis* (Chicago: AMA, 1961), 36; the same form, without the clause specifying that it is for Jewish parents, is reprinted in the 1991 edition on p. 161.

32. See William E. Brigman, "Circumcision as Child Abuse: The Legal and Constitutional Issues," *Journal of Family Law* 23 (1984–85): 337–57.

II. THE FATAL TEMPTATION: DRUG CONTROL AND SUICIDE

1. Will Rogers, "Slogans, Slogans Everywhere" [1925], in *A Will Rogers Treasury,* ed. Bryan B. and Frances N. Sterling (New York: Bonanza Books, 1982), 71.

2. "Banishing Books?" *U.S. News & World Report,* May 18, 1992, p. 76.

3. J. Somerville, "Illinois Task Force Issues Model Right-to-Die Bill," *American Medical News,* April 20, 1990, p. 20.

4. Thomas Szasz, "The Ethics of Suicide" [1971], in *The Theology of Medicine: The Political-Philosophical Foundations of Medical Ethics* [1977] (Syracuse: Syracuse University Press, 1988), 68–85.

13. PSYCHIATRY'S WAR ON CRIMINAL RESPONSIBILITY

1. For the origin of the insanity defense, see Thomas Szasz, *Fatal Freedom: The Ethics and Politics of Suicide* [1999] (Syracuse: Syracuse University Press, 2002), especially 29–44.

2. Thomas Szasz, *Insanity: The Idea and Its Consequences* [1987] (Syracuse: Syracuse University Press, 1997).

3. See Thomas Szasz, *Law, Liberty, and Psychiatry: An Inquiry into the Social Uses of Mental Health Practices* [1963] (Syracuse: Syracuse University Press, 1989); *Psychiatric Justice* [1965] (Syracuse: Syracuse University Press, 1988); and *Psychiatric Slavery: When Confinement and Coercion Masquerade as Cure* [1977] (Syracuse: Syracuse University Press, 1998).

4. "The Psychiatrist in Court: People of the State of California v. Darlin June Cromer," *American Journal of Forensic Psychiatry* 3 (1982): 5–46.

5. Ann Bancroft, "Darlin June Cromer: Three Children Testify at Murder Trial," *San Francisco Chronicle*, December 2, 1980.

6. Ibid., emphasis added.

7. P. Kuehl, "Tale of Racial Hate in Bay Murder Trial," *San Francisco Chronicle*, December 4, 1980.

8. Ibid.

9. "Jail Psychologist Testifies in Trial of Alameda Black Child's Slayer," *San Francisco Chronicle*, December 12, 1980.

10. Aric Press and Pamela Abramson, "A Law for Racist Killers," *Newsweek* (February 23, 1981): 80–81.

11. Don Martinez, "Jury Finds Cromer Guilty of Killing Boy," *San Francisco Chronicle*, January 18, 1981.

12. Ibid.

13. Don Martinez, "Testimony Winds up in Cromer Trial," *San Francisco Chronicle*, January 13, 1981, emphasis added.

14. "The Psychiatrist in Court," 9, emphasis added.

15. Ibid., 12, emphasis added.

16. Ibid., 14.

17. Ibid., 18–19, emphasis added.

18. Ibid., 19.

19. Ibid., 20–21.

20. Ibid., 26–27.

21. Seth Rosenfeld, "Conviction of Child-Killer Upheld: Woman Strangled Tot out of Racial Hatred," *San Francisco Examiner*, March 29, 1990, p. A8.

22. Nina Martin, "Conviction Challenged in 1981 Racial Slaying: Prosecutor Inflamed Jurors, Appeal Says," *San Francisco Examiner*, January 17, 1990, p. A1.

23. "The Psychiatrist in Court."

24. Ibid., 7.

25. Ibid., 35–36, emphasis added.

26. Ibid., 37, emphasis added.

27. Ibid., 44.

28. Ibid., 45–46.

29. http:// uni-wuerzburg.de/pathologie/virchow/v2/v2_kirche.htm. My translation.

30. Thomas Szasz, *Pharmacracy: Medicine and Politics in America* [2001] (Syracuse: Syracuse University Press, 2003).

14. KILLING AS THERAPY: THE CASE OF TERRI SCHIAVO

1. Quoted in Joan Didion, "The Case of Theresa Schiavo," *New York Review of Books* (June 9, 2005). For factual information about the case, see also http://www.sptimes .com/2003/webspecials03/schiavo/.

2. Ibid.

3. According to court records, Michael Schiavo did not, technically speaking, make the decision to discontinue life-prolonging measures for Terri. In 1988, after keeping Terri alive for eight years, Michael, as Terri's guardian, petitioned the Florida courts "to act as the ward's surrogate and determine what the ward would decide to do. . . . Under this procedure, the trial court becomes the surrogate decision-maker, and that is what happened in this case." The court held a trial on the dispute. Both sides presented their views and the evidence supporting those views. The trial court then determined that "the evidence showed that Terri would not wish to continue life-prolonging measures" (University of Miami Ethics Programs, "Schiavo Case Re-sources," http://www6.miami.edu/ethics2/schiavo/timeline.htm, accessed April 14, 2007).

4. An interesting mix of individuals shared the view that the court-ordered "execution" of Terri Schiavo was very wrong. Among them are former Clinton lawyer Lanny Davis, former Gore lawyer David Boies, former O. J. Simpson lawyer Alan Dershowitz, Democratic senator Joe Lieberman, civil libertarian Nat Hentoff, Green Party presidential candidate Ralph Nader, and Rainbow Coalition leader Jesse Jackson (Lifelike Pundits, "Would You Rather Be O. J.'s Girlfriend or Michael Schiavo's Fiancee?" http://www.lifelikepundits.com/archives/000519. php, March 30, 2005; accessed April 14, 2007).

5. 1 Kings 3:16–27 (King James Version).

6. Michael Schiavo quoted in http://www.sptimes.com/2003/webspecials03/schiavo/ (accessed April 14, 2007).

7. William Faulkner, "A Rose for Emily" (1935), http://xroads.virginia.edu/~drbr/wf_ rose.html (accessed April 14, 2007).

8. This phenomenon is not as rare as we might suppose. See, for example, "Man Watched TV with Dead Wife for over a Year," http://groups.google.com/group/alt.obituaries/ browse_thread/thread/4d3d4253a691a8e1/90085302327036dd%2390085302327036dd (accessed April 15, 2007).

9. Thomas Szasz, *Law, Liberty, and Psychiatry: An Inquiry into the Social Uses of Mental Health Practices* [1963] (Syracuse: Syracuse University Press, 1989).

10. Gilbert K. Chesterton, broadcast talk, June 11, 1935.

11. Thomas Szasz, *Fatal Freedom: The Ethics and Politics of Suicide* [1999] (Syracuse: Syracuse University Press, 2001).

12. "What are the admission requirements for hospice care? Consent of attending physician. Life expectancy of six months or less. Goal of comfort care rather than cure. Philosophy of allowing death to occur naturally without extraordinary intervention" (http://www.blessinghospital.org/Health%20Services/hospice%20faq.htm). "According to the Medicare hospice program, services may be provided to the terminally ill Medicare beneficiaries with a life expectancy of six months or less. However, if the patient lives beyond the initial six months, he or she can continue receiving hospice care as long as the attending physician recertifies that the patient is terminally ill. Medicare, Medicaid and many private and commercial insurers will continue to cover hospice services as long as the patient meets the criteria of having a life expectancy of six months or less" (http://www.hospicenyc .org/content/about_hospice/misconceptions.asp). Virtually the same information appears on many sites; see, for example, http://www.hospice.org/admit.htm, http://www.odyssey .net/subscribers/hospice/unyha/adcrit.html, or http://www.hospiceministriesweb.org/ admission.php.

13. Anton J. von Hooff, *From Autothanasia to Suicide: Self-Killing in Classical Antiquity* (London: Routledge, 1990), 51.

14. Thomas More, *Utopia [1516] and Other Writings* (New York: New American Library, 1984), 18.

15. Szasz, *Fatal Freedom*.

16. William Osler, "The Fixed Period," in Osler, *Aequanimitas: With Other Addresses to Medical Students, Nurses and Practitioners of Medicine*, 3rd ed. (Philadelphia: Blakiston, 1943), 375–93.

17. H. A. Johnson, "Osler Recommends Chloroform at Sixty," *Pharos* 59 (Winter 1996): 24–26.

18. Harvey Cushing, *The Life of Sir William Osler* (London: Oxford University Press, 1925), 1:669.

19. John Donne, *Biathanatos* [1646] (New York: Facsimile Text Society, 1930).

20. Anthony Trollope, *The Fixed Period* [1882] (London: Penguin, 1993).

21. Michael Schiavo quoted in Lerner, "Michael Schiavo Speaks at Local Medical Ethics Conference."

22. Thomas Friedman, "Singapore and Katrina," *New York Times,* September 14, 2005.

23. Edmund Burke, "Jacobinism" (1791), in *The Philosophy of Edmund Burke: A Selection from His Speeches and Writings,* ed. with an introduction by Louis I. Bredvold and Ralph G. Ross (Ann Arbor: University of Michigan Press, 1961), 249.

15. PETER SINGER'S ETHICS OF MEDICALIZATION

1. Peter Singer, "Philosophical Self-Portrait," in Thomas Mautner, *The Penguin Dictionary of Philosophy* (London: Penguin, 1997), 521–22. http://www.utilitarian.net/singer/by/1997——.htm.

2. Ibid.

3. Peter Singer, *Practical Ethics*, 2nd ed. (Cambridge: Cambridge University Press, 1993), 110.

4. Peter Singer, "Changing Ethics in Life and Death Decision Making," *Society* 38 (July–August 2001): 9–15.

5. Singer, *Practical Ethics*, 169–71.

6. Ibid., 186.

7. Ibid., 15.

8. Ibid., 199–200, emphasis added.

9. Gary L. Francione, "Animal Rights Theory and Utilitarianism: Relative Normative Guidance" (1997), http://www.animallaw.info/articles/arusgfrancione1997.htm (accessed April 12, 2007).

10. Thomas Szasz, *Fatal Freedom: The Ethics and Politics of Suicide* [1999] (Syracuse: Syracuse University Press, 2002).

11. Singer, "Changing Ethics in Life and Death Decision Making."

12. Jack Kevorkian, *Prescription: Medicide, The Goodness of Planned Death* (Buffalo: Prometheus Books, 1991), 202.

13. Singer, *Practical Ethics*, 329.

14. Ibid., 216, emphasis added.

15. Ibid., 218.

16. Ibid., 222.

17. Ronald Bailey, "The Pursuit of Happiness," *Reason* (December 2000), http://reason.com/0012/rb.the.shtml.

18. "Singer's Views on Disability Protested," *Minnesota Daily*, March 24, 2006. http://www.notdeadyet.org/.

19. John E. E. D. Acton, *Essays in the Study and Writing of History*, ed. J. Rufus Fears (Indianapolis: Liberty Classics, 1988), 3:572, 574.

20. Peter Bauer, in Economics Focus, "A Voice for the Poor," *Economist* (May 2, 2002).

21. Quoted in George Seldes, *The Great Quotations* (New York: Lyle Stuart, 1960), 354.

22. Peter T. Bauer, *Reality and Rhetoric: Studies in Economic Development* (London: Weidenfeld and Nicolson, 1984), 158; and Helmut Schoeck, *Envy: A Theory of Social Behaviour* [1966], trans. Michael Glenny and Betty Ross (New York: Harcourt, Brace & World, 1969).

23. Peter Singer, *Rethinking Life and Death: The Collapse of Our Traditional Ethics* (New York: St. Martin's Griffin, 1996).

24. Singer, *Practical Ethics*, 216.

25. Annie Flury, "Right to Life Challenge Goes to Court," *Times* (London), October 2, 2000, Internet edition.

26. Club of Amsterdam, "Books about the Future of Global Economy," http://www .clubofamsterdam.com/press.asp?contentid=103&catid=85 (accessed April 12, 2007).

27. Nat Hentoff, "A Professor of Infanticide at Princeton," *Jewish World Review* (September 13, 1999). http://www.jewishworldreview.com/cols/hentoff091399.asp (accessed April 15, 2007).

28. Donald Demarco, "Peter Singer: Architect of the Culture of Death," *Social Justice Review* 94 (September–October 2003): 154–57. http://www.catholiceducation.org/articles/ medical_ethics/me0049.html (accessed April 14, 2007).

29. Wesley J. Smith, *Forced Exit: The Slippery Slope from Assisted Suicide to Legalized Murder* (New York: Times Books, 1997), 21.

30. Kenneth R. Minogue, *The Liberal Mind* (London: Methuen, 1963).

31. Ibid., 7.

32. Singer, *Practical Ethics,* 275.

33. Minogue, *The Liberal Mind,* 6, emphasis in the original.

34. Ibid.

35. Ibid., 7, 10, 11, emphasis added.

36. Ibid., 8, emphasis in the original.

37. Ibid.

38. James Thomas Flexner, "He Sought to Do Good," *New York Times Book Review* (November 13, 1966): 60.

39. Acton, *Essays in the Study and Writing of History,* 3:649.

40. James Madison, "Property," in *The Writings of James Madison,* ed. Gaillard Hunt (New York: G. P. Putnam's Sons, 1900–1910), 6:101, 103, 105.

16. PHARMACRACY: THE NEW DESPOTISM

1. Steven Woloshin and Lisa M. Schwartz, "The U.S. Postal Service and Cancer Screening Stamps of Approval?" *New England Journal of Medicine* 340 (March 18, 1999): 884–87.

2. Morton H. Fried, "State: The Institution," in *International Encyclopedia of the Social Sciences,* ed. David L. Sills (New York: Macmillan and Free Press, 1968), 15:143–50, 143, 149.

3. Thomas Szasz, *Law, Liberty, and Psychiatry: An Inquiry into the Social Uses of Psychiatry* [1963] (Syracuse: Syracuse University Press, 1989); *Ceremonial Chemistry: The Ritual Persecution of Drugs, Addicts, and Pushers* [1976] (Syracuse: Syracuse University Press, 2003).

4. See the essays in this volume.

5. George Washington, http://www.brainyquote.com/quotes/authors/g/george_wash ington.html (accessed April 14, 2007).

6. Edward P. Richards and Kathrine C. Rathbun, "The Role of the Police Power in Twenty-first Century Public Health," *Sexually Transmitted Diseases* 26 (July 1999): 350–57, 356.

7. Ibid., emphasis added.

8. Robert Heinlein quoted in Bruce D. Porter, *War and the Rise of the State: The Military Foundations of Modern Politics* (New York: Free Press, 1994), xiii.

9. Robert Higgs, *Crisis and Leviathan: Critical Episodes in the Growth of American Government* (New York: Oxford University Press, 1987), 159.

10. Georges J. Danton quoted in *Bartlett's Familiar Quotations,* 16th ed., ed. Justin Kaplan (Boston: Little, Brown, 1992), 364.

11. Ibid.

12. Higgs, *Crisis and Leviathan,* x.

13. Martin van Creveld, *The Rise and Decline of the State* (Cambridge: Cambridge University Press, 1999), 7.

14. Arthur Seldon et al., *The Retreat of the State* (Norwich, U.K.: Canterbury, 2000); Susan Strange, *The Retreat of the State: The Diffusion of Power in the World Economy* (Cambridge: Cambridge University Press, 1996); Dennis Swann, *The Retreat of the State: Deregulation and Privatization in the UK and US* (Ann Arbor: University of Michigan Press, 1998).

15. Robert J. Samuelson, "Who Governs?" *Newsweek* (February 21, 2000): 33.

16. See T. Szasz, "The Therapeutic State: The Tyranny of Pharmacracy," *Independent Review* 5 (Spring 2001): 485–521.

17. James M. Buchanan, *The Limits of Liberty: Between Anarchy and Leviathan* (Chicago: University of Chicago Press, 1975), 162.

18. Thomas Szasz, *Cruel Compassion: The Psychiatric Control of Society's Unwanted* [1994] (Syracuse: Syracuse University Press, 1998), especially 150–86.

19. John Gibeaut, "Who Knows Best? It's an Ongoing Debate: Should the Government Force Treatment on the Mentally Ill?" *American Bar Association Journal* (January 2000), http://www.ptb.state.il.us/publications/Mindex-general.shtml (accessed April 14, 2007).

20. Porter, *War and the Rise of the State,* 9, emphasis added.

21. Dan E. Beauchamp, "Community: The Neglected Tradition of Public Health," in Dan E. Beauchamp and Bonnie Steinbock, eds., *New Ethics for the Public's Health* (New York: Oxford University Press, 1999), 59.

22. Geoffrey Rose, "Sick Individuals and Sick Populations," *International Journal of Epidemiology* 14 (1985): 32–38; reprinted in Beauchamp and Steinbock, eds., *New Ethics for the Public's Health,* 36–37.

23. Gerald Dworkin, "Paternalism" (1972), in Beauchamp and Steinbock, eds., *New Ethics for the Public's Health,* 127–28.

24. Alan I. Leshner quoted in David Samuels, "Saying Yes to Drugs," *New Yorker* (March 23, 1998): 48–55, 48–49.

25. Willard Gaylin and Bruce Jennings, *The Perversion of Autonomy: The Proper Uses of Coercion and Constraints in a Liberal Society* (New York: Free Press, 1996).

26. See Thomas Szasz, *Pharmacracy: Medicine and Politics in America* [2001] (Syracuse: Syracuse University Press, 2003).

27. Paul Weindling, *Health, Race, and German Politics Between National Unification and Nazism, 1870–1945* (Cambridge: Cambridge University Press, 1989), 525.

28. Ibid., 518.

29. Ibid., 544, 549, 550.

30. Ibid., 576–77, 542–43.

31. Robert N. Proctor, *The Nazi War on Cancer* (Princeton: Princeton University Press, 1999), 277.

32. Henry Friedlander, *The Origins of Nazi Genocide: From Euthanasia to the Final Solution* (Chapel Hill: University of North Carolina Press, 1995), 180–81.

33. Proctor, *The Nazi War on Cancer*, 252.

34. Ibid., 11.

35. See Szasz, *Pharmacracy*, 149.

36. Proctor, *The Nazi War on Cancer*, 136.

37. This volume, chapter 15.

38. Proctor, *The Nazi War on Cancer*, 249, 271.

39. James Fallows, "The Political Scientist: Harold Varmus Has Ambitious Plans for the Future of Medicine," *New Yorker* (June 7, 1999): 66–75, 68.

40. Richard Cobden, *The Political Writings of Richard Cobden* (1867), with a preface by Lord Welby; introductions by Sir Louis Mallet, C. B. and William Cullen Bryant; and ed. F. W. Chesson (London: T. Fisher Unwin, 1903), http://www.econlib.org/library/YPDBooks/Cobden/cbdPW7.html.

41. Roger Hayes and Emile LeBrun, "Public Health Surveillance for Firearm Injuries," *JAMA* 282 (August 4, 1999): 429–30; 429.

42. Al Gore, "Gore Sets Goal for a Cancer-Free America," http://quiz.ontheissues.org/2008/More_Al_Gore_Health_Care.htm (accessed April 14, 2007).

43. Andrew Ferguson, "What Politicians Can't Do," *Time* (May 3, 1999): 52.

Selected Bibliography

Acton, John E. E. D. *Essays in the Study and Writing of History*. Ed. J. Rufus Fears. Indianapolis: Liberty Classics, 1988.

Alexander, George J., and Alan W. Scheflin. *Law and Mental Disorder*. Durham, N.C.: Carolina Academic Press, 1998.

American Medical Association. *Medicolegal Forms with Legal Analysis*. Chicago: AMA, 1961.

American Psychiatric Association. *Diagnostic and Statistical Manual of Mental Disorders of the American Psychiatric Association (DSM-III)*. 3rd ed. Washington, D.C.: American Psychiatric Association, 1980.

———. *Diagnostic and Statistical Manual of Mental Disorders of the American Psychiatric Association (DSM-III-R)*. 3rd rev. ed. Washington, D.C.: American Psychiatric Association, 1987.

———. *DSM-IV Options Book: Work in Progress*. Washington, D.C.: American Psychiatric Association, 1991.

Bartlett's Familiar Quotations. Ed. Justin Kaplan. 16th ed. Boston: Little, Brown, 1992.

Bastiat, Frédéric. *Economic Sophisms*. 1845–48. Trans. Arthur Goddard. Princeton: Van Nostrand, 1964.

Bauer, Peter T. *Reality and Rhetoric: Studies in Economic Development*. London: Weidenfeld and Nicolson, 1984.

Beauchamp, Dan E., and Bonnie Steinbock, eds. *New Ethics for the Public's Health*. New York: Oxford University Press, 1999.

Bly, Nellie (Elizabeth Cochrane). *Ten Days in a Madhouse, or Nellie Bly's Experience on Blackwell's Island. Feigning Insanity in Order to Reveal Asylum Horrors*. New York: Norman L. Munroe, 1887.

Buchanan, James M. *The Limits of Liberty: Between Anarchy and Leviathan*. Chicago: University of Chicago Press, 1975.

Burke, Edmund. *The Philosophy of Edmund Burke: A Selection from His Speeches and Writings*. Ed. with introduction by Louis I. Bredvold and Ralph G. Ross. Ann Arbor: University of Michigan Press, 1961.

———. *Reflections on the Revolution in France*. 1790. Ed. Conor Cruise O'Brien. London: Penguin, 1986.

Chesterton, Gilbert K. *Tremendous Trifles*. New York: Dodd, Mead, 1909.

Cheyne, George. *The English Malady, Or, a Treatise of Nervous Diseases of All Kinds, as Spleen, Vapours, Lowness of Spirits, Hypochondriacal and Hysterical Distempers, etc*. London: Strahan and Leake, 1733.

Cobden, Richard. *The Political Writings of Richard Cobden*. 1867. Preface by Lord Welby; introductions by Sir Louis Mallet, C. B. and William Cullen Bryant; ed. F. W. Chesson. London: T. Fisher Unwin, 1903.

Cohen, Abraham. *Everyman's Talmud*. New York: Schocken, 1975.

Cotran, Ramzi S., Vinay Kumar, and Stanley L. Robbins. *Robbins Pathologic Basis of Disease*. 4th ed. Philadelphia: Saunders, 1989.

Crawson, R. A., et al. *Pathology: The Mechanism of Disease*. 2nd ed. Philadelphia: Mosby, 1989.

Creveld, Martin van. *The Rise and Decline of the State*. Cambridge: Cambridge University Press, 1999.

Cushing, Harvey. *The Life of Sir William Osler*. 2 vols. London: Oxford University Press, 1925.

De Duve, Christian. *Life Evolving: Molecules, Mind, and Meaning*. New York: Oxford University Press, 2002.

De Fursac, Joseph Rogues. *Manual of Psychiatry and Mental Hygiene*. 7th ed. 1903. New York: Wiley, 1938.

Dennett, D. *Consciousness Explained*. Boston: Little, Brown, 1991.

DePorte, Michael. *Nightmares and Hobbyhorses: Swift, Sterne, and Augustan Ideas of Madness*. San Marino, Calif.: Huntington Library, 1974.

Donne, John. *Biathanatos*. 1646. New York: Facsimile Text Society, 1930.

Donovan, Arthur. *Antoine Lavoisier: Science, Administration, and Revolution*. Oxford: Blackwell, 1993.

Ehrenpreis, Irwin. *Swift: The Man, His Works, and the Age*. 3 vols. Cambridge: Harvard University Press, 1983.

The Encyclopedia of Philosophy. Ed. Paul Edwards. 8 vols. New York: Macmillan and Free Press, 1967.

Engstrom, Erik J. *Clinical Psychiatry in Imperial Germany: A History of Psychiatric Practice*. Ithaca, N.Y.: Cornell University Press, 2003.

Epstein, Louis M. *Sex Laws and Customs in Judaism*. New York: Ktav Publishing House, 1967.

Feldman, David M. *Birth Control in Jewish Law: Marital Relations, Contraception, and Abortion as Set Forth in the Classical Texts of Jewish Law*. New York: New York University Press, 1968.

Foucault, Michel. *Madness and Civilization: A History of Insanity in the Age of Reason*. 1961. New York: Pantheon, 1965.

Freud, Anna. *Normality and Pathology in Childhood: Assessments of Development*. New York: International Universities Press, 1965.

Freud, Sigmund. *The Standard Edition of the Complete Psychological Works of Sigmund Freud*. Trans. James Strachey. 24 vols. London: Hogarth Press, 1953–74.

Friedlander, Henry. *The Origins of Nazi Genocide: From Euthanasia to the Final Solution*. Chapel Hill: University of North Carolina Press, 1995.

Gaylin, Willard, and Bruce Jennings. *The Perversion of Autonomy: The Proper Uses of Coercion and Constraints in a Liberal Society*. New York: Free Press, 1996.

Hawaii State Alliance for the Mentally Ill. Advertisement for "Mental Illness Awareness Week, October 6–12." *Sunday Star-Bulletin & Advertiser* (Honolulu), October 6, 1991.

Hawthorne, Nathaniel. *The Scarlet Letter*. 1850. New York: Bantam Dell, 2003.

Higgs, Robert. *Crisis and Leviathan: Critical Episodes in the Growth of American Government*. New York: Oxford University Press, 1987.

Hobbes, Thomas. *Leviathan*. Ed. M. Oakeshott. 1651. New York: Macmillan/Collier, 1962.

Hobson, Alan J. *The Chemistry of Conscious States: How The Brain Changes Its Mind*. Boston: Little, Brown, 1994.

Hooff, Anton J. van. *From Autothanasia to Suicide: Self-Killing in Classical Antiquity*. London: Routledge, 1990.

Hunter, Richard, and Ida Macalpine. *Three Hundred Years of Psychiatry, 1533–1860: A History Presented in Selected English Texts*. London: Oxford University Press, 1963.

Huxley, Aldous. *Brave New World*. 1932. New York: HarperPerennial, 1969.

International Encyclopedia of the Social Sciences. Ed. David L. Sills. New York: Macmillan and Free Press, 1968.

Kevorkian, Jack. *Prescription: Medicide, The Goodness of Planned Death*. Buffalo: Prometheus Books, 1991.

Keynes, John M. *The Economic Consequences of the Peace*. Introduction by Robert Lekachman. 1920. New York: Penguin, 1970.

Kierkegaard, Søren. *Parables of Kierkegaard*. Ed. Thomas C. Oden. Princeton: Princeton University Press, 1978.

Kissane, John M., ed. *Anderson's Pathology*. 9th ed. Philadelphia: Mosby, 1990.

Kraepelin, Emil. *Einführung in die psychiatrische Klinik*. Leipzig: Johann Ambrosius Barth, 1901.

———. *Lectures on Clinical Psychiatry*. 1901. New York: Hafner, 1968.

Krafft-Ebing, Richard von. *Psychopathia Sexualis, with Special Reference to the Antipathic Sexual Instinct: A Medico-Forensic Study*. 1886. Authorized English adaptation of the 12th German edition by F. J. Rebman, rev. ed. Brooklyn, N.Y.: Physicians and Surgeons Book Company, 1931.

Lewis, Clive S. *Mere Christianity*. New York: Macmillan, 1952.

Madison, James. *The Writings of James Madison*. Ed. Gaillard Hunt. 9 vols. New York: G. P. Putnam's Sons, 1900–1910.

Maimonides, Moses. *The Guide for the Perplexed*. New York: Dover, 1956.

Masters, William, and Virginia Johnson. *Human Sexual Inadequacy*. Boston: Little, Brown, 1970.

Mautner, Thomas. *The Penguin Dictionary of Philosophy*. London: Penguin, 1997.

McElrath, Damien. *Lord Acton: The Decisive Decade, 1864–1874; Essays and Documents*. Louvain, Belgium: Publications Universitaires de Louvain, 1970.

Minogue, Kenneth R. *The Liberal Mind*. London: Methuen, 1963.

Money, A. *Treatment of Disease in Children*. Philadelphia: Blakiston, 1887.

More, Thomas. *Utopia [1516] and Other Writings*. New York: New American Library, 1984.

O'Donoghue, E. G. *The Story of Bethlehem Hospital, From Its Foundation in 1247*. New York: Dutton, 1915.

Osler, William. *Aequanimitas: With Other Addresses to Medical Students, Nurses, and Practitioners of Medicine*. 3rd ed. Philadelphia: Blakiston, 1943.

Paige, Karen E., and Jeffrey M. Paige. *The Politics of Reproductive Ritual*. Berkeley: University of California Press, 1981.

Parry-Jones, William L. *The Trade in Lunacy: A Study of Private Madhouses in England in the Eighteenth and Nineteenth Centuries*. London: Routledge and Kegan Paul, 1976.

Plato. *Republic*. Trans. Paul Shorey. In *The Collected Dialogues of Plato, Including the Letters*. Ed. Edith Hamilton and Huntington Cairns. Princeton: Princeton University Press, 1961.

Polanyi, Michael. *Knowing and Being: Essays by Michael Polanyi*. Ed. Marjorie Grene. Chicago: University of Chicago Press, 1969.

Boston Public Library

Customer ID: **************7367**

Title: The medicalization of everyday life
ID: 39999052479258
Due: 04/10/12

Total items: 1
3/20/2012 4:54 PM

Thank you for using the
3M SelfCheck™ System.

Porter, Bruce D. *War and the Rise of the State: The Military Foundations of Modern Politics.* New York: Free Press, 1994.

Porter, Roy. *Flesh in the Age of Reason: The Modern Foundations of Body and Soul.* New York: Norton, 2004.

————. *Mind-Forg'd Manacles: A History of Madness from the Restoration to the Regency.* London: Athlone Press, 1987.

Priestley, Joseph. *Considerations on the Doctrine of Phlogiston and the Decomposition of Water.* Philadelphia: Thomas Dobson, 1796.

Proctor, Robert N. *The Nazi War on Cancer.* Princeton: Princeton University Press, 1999.

Remondino, Peter C. *History of Circumcision: From the Earliest Times to the Present.* Philadelphia: F. A. Davis, 1891. Reprint; New York: AMS Press, 1974.

Reynolds, E. H., and M. R. Trimble, eds. *Epilepsy and Psychiatry.* London: Churchill Livingstone, 1981.

Rogers, Will. *A Will Rogers Treasury: Reflections and Observations.* Ed. Bryan B. and Frances N. Sterling. New York: Bonanza Books, 1982.

Romains, Jules. *Knock, ou le triomphe de médecine.* Trans. James B. Gidney. 1923. Great Neck, N.Y.: Barron Educational Series, 1962.

Rubin, Emanuel, and John L. Farber, eds. *Pathology.* Philadelphia: Lippincott, 1988.

Rush, Benjamin. *Medical Inquiries and Observations Upon the Diseases of the Mind.* 1812. New York: Macmillan-Hafner Press, 1962.

Russell, Bertrand. *A History of Western Philosophy: And Its Connection with Political and Social Circumstances from the Earliest Times to the Present Day.* New York: Simon and Schuster, 1945.

————. *Sceptical Essays.* London: Allen and Unwin, 1928.

Ryle, Gilbert. *The Concept of Mind.* London: Hutchinson's University Library, 1949.

Schoeck, Helmut. *Envy: A Theory of Social Behaviour.* Trans. Michael Glenny and Betty Ross. 1966. New York: Harcourt, Brace and World, 1969.

Schreber, Daniel. *Memoirs of My Nervous Illness.* Trans. Ida Macalpine and Richard Hunter. 1903. London: William Dawson and Sons, 1955.

Seldes, George. *The Great Quotations.* New York: Lyle Stuart, 1960.

Seldon, Arthur, et al. *The Retreat of the State.* Norwich, U.K.: Canterbury, 2000.

Singer, Peter. *Practical Ethics.* 2nd ed. Cambridge: Cambridge University Press, 1993.

————. *Rethinking Life and Death: The Collapse of Our Traditional Ethics.* New York: St. Martin's Griffin, 1996.

Smith, Wesley J. *Forced Exit: The Slippery Slope from Assisted Suicide to Legalized Murder*. New York: Times Books, 1997.

Strange, Susan. *The Retreat of the State: The Diffusion of Power in the World Economy*. Cambridge: Cambridge University Press, 1996.

Swann, Dennis. *The Retreat of the State: Deregulation and Privatization in the UK and US*. Ann Arbor: University of Michigan Press, 1998.

Swift, Jonathan. *The Examiner*, no. 15 (November 9, 1710). http://www.ourcivilisation.com/smartboard/shop/swift/examiner/chap14.htm (accessed April 15, 2007).

———. *Jonathan Swift*. Ed. A. Ross and D. Woolley. New York: Oxford University Press, 1984.

Szasz, Thomas. *Anti-Freud: Karl Kraus's Criticism of Psychoanalysis and Psychiatry*. 1976. Syracuse: Syracuse University Press, 1990.

———. *Ceremonial Chemistry: The Ritual Persecution of Drugs, Addicts, and Pushers*. 1976. Syracuse: Syracuse University Press, 2003.

———. *Cruel Compassion: The Psychiatric Control of Society's Unwanted*. 1994. Syracuse: Syracuse University Press, 1998.

———. *The Ethics of Psychoanalysis: The Theory and Method of Autonomous Psychotherapy*. 1965. Syracuse: Syracuse University Press, 1988.

———. *Fatal Freedom: The Ethics and Politics of Suicide*. 1999. Syracuse: Syracuse University Press, 2002.

———. *Ideology and Insanity: Essays on the Psychiatric Dehumanization of Man*. 1970. Syracuse: Syracuse University Press, 1991.

———. *Insanity: The Idea and Its Consequences*. 1987. Syracuse: Syracuse University Press, 1997.

———. *Law, Liberty, and Psychiatry: An Inquiry into the Social Uses of Psychiatry*. 1963. Syracuse: Syracuse University Press, 1989.

———. *A Lexicon of Lunacy: Metaphoric Malady, Moral Responsibility, and Psychiatry*. New Brunswick, N.J.: Transaction Publishers, 1993.

———. *Liberation By Oppression: A Comparative Study of Slavery and Psychiatry*. New Brunswick, N.J.: Transaction Publishers, 2002.

———. *The Manufacture of Madness: A Comparative Study of the Inquisition and the Mental Health Movement*. 1970. Syracuse: Syracuse University Press, 1997.

———. *The Meaning of Mind: Language, Morality, and Neuroscience*. 1996. Syracuse: Syracuse University Press, 2002.

———. *The Myth of Mental Illness: Foundations of a Theory of Personal Conduct*. 1961. Rev. ed. New York: HarperCollins, 1974.

———. *The Myth of Psychotherapy: Mental Healing as Religion, Rhetoric, and Repression*. 1978. Syracuse: Syracuse University Press, 1988.

———. *Our Right to Drugs: The Case for a Free Market*. 1992. Syracuse: Syracuse University Press, 1996.

———. *Pain and Pleasure: A Study of Bodily Feelings*. 1957. 2nd expanded ed. 1975. Syracuse: Syracuse University Press, 1988.

———. *Pharmacracy: Medicine and Politics in America*. 2001. Syracuse: Syracuse University Press, 2003.

———. *Psychiatric Justice*. 1965. Syracuse: Syracuse University Press, 1988.

———. *Psychiatric Slavery: When Confinement and Coercion Masquerade as Cure*. 1977. Syracuse: Syracuse University Press, 1998.

———. *Schizophrenia: The Sacred Symbol of Psychiatry*. 1976. Syracuse: Syracuse University Press, 1988.

———. *The Second Sin*. Garden City, N.Y.: Doubleday Anchor, 1973.

———. *Sex by Prescription: The Startling Truth about Today's Sex Therapy*. 1980. Syracuse: Syracuse University Press, 1990.

———. *The Theology of Medicine: The Political-Philosophical Foundations of Medical Ethics*. 1977. Syracuse: Syracuse University Press, 1988.

———. *The Therapeutic State: Psychiatry in the Mirror of Current Events*. Buffalo: Prometheus Books, 1984.

———. *Words to the Wise: A Medical-Philosophical Dictionary*. New Brunswick, N.J.: Transaction, 2003.

Szasz, Thomas., ed. *The Age of Madness: A History of Involuntary Mental Hospitalization Presented in Selected Texts*. Garden City, N.Y.: Doubleday Anchor, 1973.

Trollope, Anthony. *The Fixed Period*. 1882. London: Penguin, 1993.

Wallerstein, Edward. *Circumcision: An American Health Fallacy*. New York: Springer, 1980.

Weindling, Paul. *Health, Race, and German Politics Between National Unification and Nazism, 1870–1945*. Cambridge: Cambridge University Press, 1989.

Wodehouse, P. G. *The Inimitable Jeeves*. 1923. London: Penguin Books, 1999.

Wormuth, Francis D. *The Origins of Modern Constitutionalism*. New York: Harper and Row, 1949.

Index